"Walk Yourself Well is the owner's manual for self-healing.
Everyone on two feet should have this book."
—Larry Payne, Ph.D., chairman, International Association
of Yoga Therapists, and co-author of *Yoga for Dummies*

"What Sherry Brourman has taught me is invaluable. She's
achieved a shared level of consciousness which has allowed me
greater insight into not only how I manage my back but also
how I move through and take care of my body. Her instruction in
corrective walking put me back on my feet stronger and wiser. She
is the most creative physical therapist I have ever met."
—Paul Michael Glaser, director and actor

"Fearing disc surgery, I was fortunate to find Sherry Brourman,
with whose guidance my back was healed in a few weeks. But
more importantly, she gave me a new relationship to my own
body which was like being reintroduced to an old friend. The
simple principles which underlie her approach—here codified in
entertaining, lucid prose—are both empowering and significant in
unexpected ways. For what Sherry really has to teach is that we
become what we practice, be it physically in the way we move or,
by implication, in the way we imagine ourselves."
—Daniel Attias, film and television writer/director

"Her explanations are clear enough for any health professional to
follow and use, and yet very understandable, even enjoyable, for the
layman. Do not be misled by the clarity and simplicity of this
method; its results are profound."
—Eddy Rosen, P.T.

"Ms. Brourman has given us a very personal and holistic account of
how poor function is the hidden cause of most chronic pain. Most
importantly, she shows the how-to of taking an active role in
addressing this dysfunction."
—Craig Liebenson, D.C.

WALK YOURSELF WELL

ELIMINATE BACK, NECK, SHOULDER, KNEE, HIP, AND OTHER STRUCTURAL PAIN FOREVER—WITHOUT SURGERY OR DRUGS

Sherry Brourman, P.T.

with Randy Rodman

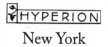

New York

All matters regarding your health require medical supervision. Consult your physician before adopting the treatment suggestions in this book, as well as about any condition that may require diagnosis or medical attention.

Library of Congress Cataloging-in-Publication Data

Brourman, Sherry
Walk yourself well : eliminate back, shoulder, knee, hip, and other structural pain forever, without surgery or drugs / by Sherry Brourman, with Randy Rodman.
p. cm.

Includes index.
ISBN 0-7868-6293-9
1. Gait disorders—Exercise therapy.   2. Gait disorders—
Complications.   3. Gait in humans.   I. Rodman, Randy
II. Title.
RC376.5.B76   1998
616.7'062—dc21   97-17885
CIP

Paperback ISBN 0-7868-8362-6

Designed by Chris Welch
First edition

10   9   8   7   6   5   4   3   2   1

IMPORTANT NOTE TO READERS

If you are in pain, please see Appendix C to establish precisely what your level of discomfort is. Your pain may fluctuate, but the scale will provide you with a reference point for the seriousness of your condition. If you are above level five in pain, and the program offered in this book does not reduce your soreness at least sometimes, then you need outside help. If you can't find a few positions in which to read this book comfortably, then you need outside help, too.

I have worked with brilliant doctors, chiropractors, acupuncturists, Rolfers, therapists, and other professionals who create wonderful results for their patients. This book will help you know when you're in the right hands and when you're not. Much of this book is about learning to trust your intuition and taking control of your own well-being.

The material in this book is for informational purposes only and is not intended to replace the advice of your health care practitioners. Please discuss any pain you're experiencing with them before beginning this program. If you have any preexisting medical conditions, or are taking any prescription or nonprescription medications, consult with your health care practitioner before beginning this program or altering or discontinuing use of any medication.

ACKNOWLEDGEMENTS

To do something innovative in a world that is doing all it can to provide obstacles or force you to conform takes unreasonable amounts of support and love. I am very blessed with both.

I would like to thank:

For the focused quiet clarity he has and gives, my partner, David Alden. His patience, generosity, and unbelievable flexibility were daily doses of strength and courage.

For the huge growth he was forced to take on in order to help me get this done, my precious son, Keith Michael Gould. His love, honesty, and depth challenged and taught me in ever-brightening ways.

My Mother, Liz Brourman, who handed me the football, knowing I would run.

My Father, Philip Brourman, and stepmother, Judy Brourman, who show me that the art of personal growth never stops.

My sisters, Michele Brourman Silas, Robin Brourman Munson, and Nancy Ziskind Hittman, who are constantly reminding me that love, trust, and growth can translate into courage, persistence, and accomplishment.

My friend, my voice, my collaborator, Randy Rodman, who stepped into this project when it was fragile and breathed strength and, best of all, fun into the process and the text.

Kristin Kliemann and the entire Hyperion family, whose faith, brilliance, and warmth have allowed this book to be in perfect balance.

April Foss, my office cohort, amazing therapist, solid friend, whose respect and reliability have given me strength through otherwise impossible times.

Mya Zapata, Lisa Coleman, and Jonathan Zapala, my office, no, my life angels.

And a special thanks to Mya, wise beyond her years and for my daily Rose.

Jonathan Kirsch, my friend and attorney, who helped me stay peaceful and passionate about this process.

Robert Tabian, my agent and seer, whose broad spectrum about this project never stopped growing.

My dear friend Sara Charno, who helped me write the first outline for this book and who continues to help the Universe help me, in her own gentle way.

Larry Payne, for so many years of inspiration, validation, support, and friendship.

Benjamin Shield, for guiding me through every phase of this book, including giving me the courage to let it be finished.

Eddy Rosen, for his time, age-old love, and gifted expertise, in my final read.

Paul Michael Glaser, who is my best fan and dear friend.

Carla Baron, for busting me and teaching me to be real.

Robert Levine, CPA, for his patience and calm judgment over my weakest link.

Tamara Atkins Conley, for casting her loving spell on the mail that day and generally being the good witch of the north.

Tammy Boe Swan, impeccable assistant therapist and friend, for being "on call" for years.

Alix Evans and Jennifer Welsh, whose time, love, energy, and corrections made this manuscript an easier read.

Drs. Jon Greenfield, Rene Cailliet, Michael Sinel, Steve Brourman, Steve Rabin, and my lifesaver, Jeffry Rush, who have been such wonderful support for my clinic.

Richard Robertson, for being a friend for all of us, through thick and thin.

Claudio Lazo, my friend and photographer, for making "pretty" feel easy.

Gady Hakim, my illustrator, for persisting through nearly insurmountable obstacles.

Patricia Reopel, who helped me build the foundation for a decade.

Jay DeCosio, who helped me name my system.

If I could, I would name every one of the instrumental teachers and angels I have been blessed with and that would be a very long list. Please know that I remember and thank you all.

CONTENTS

INTRODUCTION

Nothing can unravel the quality of your life faster than pain. It is our birthright to grow, experience, achieve, and enjoy life without painful physical distraction. This book provides a tested system for realigning and healing your body to eliminate and prevent physical discomfort and suffering.

Although it seems that walking correctly should be something everybody does automatically, it's not. When I visit New York City, or any time I have an opportunity to watch a lot of people walk, I am struck by the urge to tell many of them that they could prevent impending structural damage, or eliminate pain, if they just made a few simple corrections to the way they walk. *Walk Yourself Well* is the first book that teaches the art of walking as an integral part of physical well-being.

Besides the fact that changing the way you walk can absolutely eliminate structural pain, I focus on walking for two reasons. First, people walk more than any other physical activity. Walking defines most everything about you, including your predisposition to pain, your athletic prowess, and your health with respect to aging. Second, walking is a universal exercise that many, including myself, consider a meditative act. No matter what's happening in my life, when I need a new perspective, I can walk to find answers. Generations of people have found the spiritual and meditative benefits of walking.

As a professional physical therapist with twenty-five years of experience, I've treated all types of pain, and I know how compelling it is to be able to move around comfortably. Several years ago I was a patient myself, struck by a condition that caused me extreme pain in my lower back, the type of pain that prevented me from moving. Several well-respected orthopedic doctors told me I needed spinal surgery. Instead, I recovered completely using the methods described in this book. At my clinic, our patients learn to incorporate this same system to eliminate their own pain.

At my clinic, I often encounter layers of mental reluctance and physical resistance that make the process harder than it really is. Old habits die hard, even when they're detrimental to your health. If you can understand that this is a process, one that will be served well by taking your time and going step-by-step, your physical and mental barriers to healing will fall away, as will your backaches, swollen joints, neck soreness, and a myriad of other problems. It's an inexpensive, drug-free, and surgery-free method of ending nagging pain, even if the pain has been with you for years. The methods in this book involve an evolutionary approach to movement that can enable you to stand up strong and live freer of pain for the rest of your life.

MY PERSONAL EXPERIENCE WITH PAIN

It was an orthopedic doctor friend who first pointed out my problem. At a swimming party, he looked at my back and blithely commented, "Sherry, I'll be doggoned if you don't have a spondy." "Spondy" is short for spondylolisthesis, and it means that a vertebra in your spine has slipped forward.

It could have been a minor birth defect that left me without one of those little hook gizmos called facets that are designed to keep vertebrae in line. Or maybe I snapped it off as I fell ice-skating or horseback riding. They're so tiny, it would be easy to crack one and not know it. My doctor friend thought that mine was never there to begin with. As a result, my lowest vertebra slid inward just enough for him to observe a small dimple or indentation on my lower back where there should have been a little extrusion.

I knew this doctor through my work as a physical therapist and I respected his opinion, so we went to the office to take an X ray, and sure enough, I had a spondy. He told me that if I didn't fall hard on it (that is, if I stopped skiing, horseback riding, and skating) and didn't have a car accident or deliver a child, I could remain pain-free for my whole life.

Well, I couldn't give up everything. I managed to cut down on horseback riding, but I couldn't do without ice-skating and skiing. And my datebook made no mention of having planned the car accident—or my baby, for that matter. And yet even after I did most of the things I was warned against, I remained pain-free: healthy, fit, and active. I approached life with innocent abandon, confident that my body would continue to perform for me.

Years later, about six months after my son, Keith, was born, I had my first big night out. I zipped myself into my favorite jeans (they finally fit again) and went out dancing. I came home and went to sleep. A few hours later I was awakened by a pain in my back so severe that it felt like a knife was sticking deep into my spine. I gasped in pain. Everything I did hurt. Simply to move, turn to my side, or sit up, shot pain through my entire body.

Walking was nearly impossible. My top half felt disconnected from my bottom half. When I curled up into a ball, the pain subsided, but then uncurling was so terrible that it wasn't worth it.

I felt absolutely shattered, powerless, exhausted, horrified, and angry at this surprise attack. I needed to get a grip and steer myself away from the agony. I wanted to know what had happened so I could choose a corrective course of action. I was desperate to stop the appalling pain.

I went to several extremely well respected doctors for their medical opinions. All of them said that I needed surgery to have my spine fused. Some of them said I needed it immediately, or my spine could break the next time I experienced any form of impact.

There I was, an accomplished physical therapist with years of expertise in virtually all areas of physical rehabilitation and pain, and my options seemed narrowed down to surgery. How ironic for me to be in this predicament.

I contemplated the situation deeply. My inner voice told me to seek another path, something other than major surgery. I couldn't afford to be down for that long, and having watched several of those surgeries, and seeing the often futile results, the concept was utterly disturbing. Unfortunately, everything I knew as a physical therapist appeared to be inadequate to provide me with the relief I desperately needed.

INTEGRATING A PLAN FOR PERSONAL SURVIVAL

The year I found out about my spondy, I had just made a big career move. I'd joined two highly qualified orthopedic surgeons. I established and ran a private physical therapy clinic for them. Frequently watching these highly respected doctors perform surgery, and dealing with their patients who suffered from chronic pain, gave me extremely valuable information about orthopedic medicine.

Long-term rehabilitation patients, like the ones I treated for years, are different from orthopedic patients. Rehabilitation patients are often accident victims who are hit with sudden trauma and instantaneous disabilities. Pain is not the issue as much as the disability, and rehab patients are anxious to recover and get on with their lives. They usually become modestly optimistic about their prognosis.

On the other hand, orthopedic patients who have suffered with pain for a long time, the ones whose disabilities don't show, often believe they will never be free of pain again. They aren't scared; they're angry. They have a short fuse, and sometimes their best mood is grumpy.

In terms of dealing with people who live in pain, I had experienced just about everything. So I thought. I was about to experience a whole new type of patient: the scariest of them all—the one I found in myself.

Despair is a grisly form of powerlessness that I refused to accept. I was not going to surrender to pain or to an intimidating surgery. The alternative became clear when I met a neurosurgeon named Ron Lawrence. Dr. Lawrence was the first highly qualified expert I talked to who seemed as uninspired with surgery as I was. He agreed that choosing surgery was premature, further adding that I was "too fit and too knowledgeable about the human body to surrender to anything that permanent." He recommended that I strengthen my abdomen muscles, not wear heels of any kind, and swim every day, or else I really would be headed for spinal surgery.

In formulating my own recovery program, my first priority was to reduce the pain. I learned by experimenting that squeezing my belly really tight before I changed positions prevented pain. But I really had to squeeze like crazy before I moved, or else I would get a shot of pain that took my breath away. I used every exercise I knew to strengthen myself. I used stretching exercises too, but anything that bent my torso forward only felt good momentarily. I'd get stuck that way and have to wiggle and jiggle myself straight again.

These types of positions are called comfort zones. A comfort zone is any position or movement that takes pain away, but only temporarily, and without any long-term healing benefits. People often feel even worse following comfort zone movements because they can aggravate injuries and/or lengthen the healing process by overstretching weakened joints, muscles, and ligaments. It took me a while to realize this, and unknowingly I made my situation worse.

My situation was compounded by something else. I thought that my sole problem was a faulty lower spine. It wasn't; my lower spine was simply my weakest link. If I had recognized and treated that weak link earlier, I could have prevented the pain before it started. Instead, *I walked right into it.*

Since my background was in long-range, extensive rehabilitative treatment of more permanent injuries and illnesses, that was how I approached my own problem. Yet I needed a fast-acting remedy more typical of orthopedic treatment. All I knew was that I was prepared to take on the most instrumental project of my life. I proceeded to integrate rehabilitation therapy with the orthopedic remedy I desperately needed.

At the time, I had no mental image of changing the way I walked, or the way I leaned back, or how I locked my knees with each step. My goal was to stop the pain. To do that, I began trying numerous exercises and positions from my past experience. I made up new ones by sensing what helped. I tried every theoretical resource and wild gimmick I could think of to keep from hurting. Then I would evaluate what worked and what didn't.

I studied and recorded which motions contained therapeutic (long-term) benefits versus just getting me into another comfort zone. I drew a quick connection between reduced pain and a change of posture. I confirmed that squeezing my belly when I changed positions always reduced my pain significantly, and that a light but constant abdominal squeezing helped in general. However, this was extremely difficult to keep up indefinitely. If I forgot, or if I accidentally lay on my stomach for more than a minute, or if I twisted a certain way, I'd get a shot of pain that might last for days.

During this excruciating period, my body seemed to contort out of control. I'd go into a weird sideways position that decreased my ability to squeeze my abdomen. That meant no progress—and more pain. So when I recovered to a point where I could resume my strengthening exercises, I used every second, every step, every movement as an opportunity to strengthen. No matter what I was doing, from washing dishes to getting dressed, I worked my muscles full-time.

I learned that when my belly was taut, I was naturally more forward on my feet, with less weight on my heels. As soon as I released my belly muscles, I'd go back on my heels and would suddenly relapse into pain. The two went hand in hand. So I intentionally stayed forward as a habit, which forced me to keep my belly and back muscles performing in unison. This action of squeezing my stomach and back muscles together as a means of generating musculoskeletal stability (which I later would come to call the "sandwich system") provided the structural stability I needed for my spine. The more they worked together, the less pain I had. I could see that this happened in parallel with standing up straight.

When I was hurting, I walked around looking like I'd just been shot in the back with an arrow. With practice, however, I was able to move around like a normal human being. Once my pain was finally under control, I decided it was time to go to work again.

I got a part-time job doing physical therapy for a doctor who ultimately fired me when he learned that I told his neck patients to run for their lives before he tractioned them into needing surgery. He had a primitive traction setup, and no clue as to the angles at which to pull the patient's head or how many pounds of pressure to use. But during this period my back situation stabilized thoroughly. I was even well enough to teach an aerobics class. I could avoid pain by staying forward on my feet and squeezing my belly. So I walked differently, and I held myself with more strength when I moved.

I traversed both ends of the emotional spectrum, being hugely pleased with my self-healing but shocked at the limited thinking and medical mismanagement I'd seen. This horrific, yet enlightening, experience fueled my desire to help others. I became more passionate about incorporating safe, practical, proven methods of pain treatment.

My recovery was not miraculous, nor was it accomplished overnight. It took time and effort. But it was absolutely thorough, and I was determined to teach other people how to live without pain. I finally opened my own physical therapy clinic.

ONE SIZE FITS ALL

One of my first patients was Stephanie. Stephanie was thirty-eight years old when she smashed up her VW. She got smashed up in the process, too. Her wounds healed, but she complained of constant back and shoulder pain months after the accident.

Stephanie leaned back when she walked, and had done so since she was a kid. As a result, her back and belly muscles were weak. As a sound engineer, working at a mixing board, Stephanie perched on a little stool most of the day. She did a lot of slouching when she sat, which further weakened her back and belly muscles. Holding her right arm out at the sound board put constant strain on her right shoulder. All this led to weak links in her lower back and her right shoulder. Then she had the car accident.

I spent some time thinking about Stephanie's structural deficiencies in the context of her shoulder pain. I could see that her back and belly muscles were extremely weak, but I didn't know that a weak trunk could cause vulnerability in someone's shoulder. I treated her back and shoulder pain as separate entities.

Although her back problem was not like mine, I was confident that strengthening her abdomen would prove beneficial. So I put her on an exercise program, the same one that took me months to develop for my own survival. I taught her the techniques I'd used to heal myself.

As her treatment progressed, I learned more about Stephanie's posture, such as how she sat at work. I determined that she had a pre-existing problem with her back and right shoulder. As is often the case, the accident aggravated a vulnerable situation.

The thrilling part for me was watching her pain shrink while she was using my strengthening system. To see it work on someone with a totally different back problem, with tangential benefits to her shoulder, was absolutely exhilarating. Stephanie's first big pain breakthrough came as the result of implementing the same system that had worked for me: her abdomen and back muscles strengthened and sandwiched her spine and lower torso together, which helped her to balance properly.

SYMPTOM THERAPY VERSUS SOURCE THERAPY

After Stephanie's success, I tried variations with other patients. I learned what worked best for which types of problems. The corresponding treatment would either corroborate my techniques or give me new information upon which I continued to build.

I began to realize that I was developing a new form of physical therapy that was both effective and rather nonconformist. My system is based on rehabilitative concepts—diagonals, quadrants, and movement patterns—that treat the body as a unit. It questions *why* a vulnerability exists and goes beyond treating the symptoms. My techniques largely deal with the way you walk—which is also called your gait—and use corresponding strengthening and stretching exercises. This has worked with profound success. Every single day at my clinic, people experience dramatic improvements.

Surgery is not an easy option. It works quickly and directly, but it often misses the underlying cause. If you looked at one hundred spinal MRIs of normal people, about seventy-five of them would show some evidence of a slipped or defective disk. Out of those, fifty patients would be asymptomatic (that is, they would experience no pain). So damaged disks are not always the underlying cause, and even when they are, most of the time damaged disks are the result of being out of balance. Achieving balanced movement is the correct starting point for most disk-related damage.

Because healed patients rarely repeat their MRI scans, we don't know if their disks have been repaired or if instead the muscles and ligaments around them have strengthened and thus stabilized the weakened area. Unfortunately, many people still think surgery is the most technologically advanced approach and the best our medical community has to offer. That concept is worth rethinking.

The other popular alternatives are not very refreshing either: drugs, total immobility (or bed rest), using braces, and therapy aimed at the symptom instead of the cause. These passive pain treatments are often as inappropriate as surgery and can be counterproductive.

The problem is that both surgery and medicine address only the parts of the body that are in pain, rather than what caused the pain in the first place. Symptomatic treatment is not the best answer for most structural pain of the back, neck, shoulder, hip, knee, and ankle. Source therapy is a better alternative because it traces pain beyond the symptomatic weak link to the cause. Source therapy also rallies the resources of the entire body to support the recovery.

Over the past five years, I've dedicated much of my time to figuring out a way to help people without the necessity of an office visit. My patients incessantly tell me to publish my system. So I've taken the system, which I call "Primary Movement Balancing," and reworked it into a format that can be taught without my personal diagnosis or private contact. This book is the result. It will enable you to customize your own personal program according to your body, your schedule, and your specific pain.

My fondest dream is that this book will become a preventative tool, rather than just a means of making body repairs. I hope that one day health care providers, insurance companies, and everyone else will realize that preventative measures can reduce structural weakness and thus decrease the frequency and intensity of injuries. Fortunately, your individual initiative has gotten you this far. Understanding the principles contained in this book, and following the simple instructions and exercises, will change your life forever. Every step you take can be a strengthening one, walking away from pain.

Note: The terminology used throughout this book has been simplified. Your quadriceps femoris, for example, is referred to as your thigh muscle. But for those who appreciate anatomical nomenclature—and the exactness it provides in locating specific body parts—we've included some technical terms on occasion, too. All muscles referred to in this book are illustrated in Appendix B (page 269).

> Thoughout this book you'll encounter text inside boxes like this one, which provides a technical explanation and greater detail to the topic at hand.

≋ 1 ≋

You Walked into Pain

How Walking with Imbalance Absolutely Leads to Pain

Walking into pain is not like walking into a wall. It's worse. When it's you versus the wall, the injury is quick. You dust yourself off and, ideally, improve your future method of navigation. When it's you versus the way you walk, however, the injury is insidious and powerful. One minor posture error repeated millions of times can do an incredible amount of damage to your muscles, nerves, and bones, eventually causing incredible pain.

This book is about fixing pain by correcting the motion you repeat most often: walking. Because the way you walk is perceived as an inherited trait, something immutable, or genetically fixed, your first reaction may be to doubt that anyone can change it. But even though genetics is a factor, it has relatively little to do with how you walk today. You learned it, and you can change it.

Eliminating pain, however, isn't the only benefit you'll derive by balancing the way you walk. These corrections improve muscle tone and enhance your overall physical appearance. Your strengths, your contours, and your overall shape are the result of repeated movements—or lack thereof. It's no mystery that usage tightens, disuse loosens. So you may end up losing inches after using this system. But the primary intentions of this book are to release your body of pain and to reduce your potential for future injuries. You'll accomplish this by balancing your body. You will eliminate structural weaknesses— weaknesses you walked into without even knowing it—from head to toes.

PRIMARY MOVEMENT PATTERNS

Have you ever sat down with a cup of tea and pondered the way you walk? If your style of walking gets you around adequately, probably not. Nevertheless, you have a walk all your own, your Primary Movement Pattern (PMP). Your walk involves thousands of body parts, all interacting to produce your style of head carriage, shoulder twist, arm swing, hip movement, knee action, and the way you plant your foot. It's as natural to you as breathing or blinking, and it probably came to you without any form of conscious planning. The way you walk may not be altogether unique, at least not like a fingerprint or voiceprint, but to a trained eye your walk is filled with distinctive characteristics that tell a story about where you have pain or where you may soon develop pain.

At the gym, most people see outfits, or buns, or glistening muscles. Not that these things escape my attention entirely, but what I tend to see are lines and angles. In kinesiological terms, I see "lever arms." When I notice someone particularly graceful or strong, or both, I enjoy observing the lines and angles that make such movement possible. At sporting events, when I see an athlete struggle, I can usually gather clues as to why: a forward head, a tendency to lean back, shoulders that roll forward, knees that lock, and so on.

The beach provides an observational gallery virtually unparalleled for PMP spectating. Among the many things sunbathers tend to expose are the bottoms of their feet, which present a self-contained catalog of a person's Primary Movement Pattern. It's not that I actually walk up to people and check out the bottoms of their feet, but if I did, I might notice that someone's heel callus is pushed over more to the inside or more to the outside. This indicates that the person's heel strike (where the heel first touches the ground) is on the side, where the callus is least pronounced.

If your heel callus is pushed to the inside, it's certain that your footprint in the sand would reveal that the outside of your foot goes deepest. If your heel callus is pushed more toward the outside, then the opposite is true. If you have your socks off and are waving your feet in the air trying to scrutinize your calluses, don't. We haven't gotten to the part of the book where you analyze your gait yet. But you will become more aware of foot pronation (rolling your foot inward when you walk) because it plays an important role in determining your PMP. And this can indicate whether or not you're a likely candidate for knee problems, lower back pain, and/or neck or shoulder injuries.

The way you walk is the foundation of your Primary Movement Pattern. Your PMP involves more than your gait, though. It shows itself in every move you make. When you sit down on a park bench, pick up the Sunday newspaper, reach for a beer mug off the top shelf, or just stand still to chat about the neighbor's funny Chihuahua, your PMP is shining through. You take this deeply ingrained pattern with you throughout your life. Your gait coalesces your PMP history into a grand finale. Your gait also maps out where and how your pain is likely to surface first. If your gait is derived from strength and balance, those qualities will be reflected in every move you make. If your gait has deviated from symmetry and balance, the rest of your motions will have, too. And if so, you've probably developed corresponding weaknesses and focal points of stress that may lead to breakdown and pain.

Y O U R　B O D Y ' S　W E A K　L I N K

The most widespread disorder in the world is structural pain—pain caused by the misalignment of the body. Backaches are the most common, followed in order by neck, shoulder, hip, knee, and ankle pain. Sometimes the misalignment can be traced directly to the way you walk. Sometimes the way you walk can be the result of some preexisting misalignment. It's like the question about the chicken or the egg, except which came first isn't that important. Your pain is.

Unless you have a naturally balanced posture and gait, you have already developed a structural vulnerability. That vulnerability may remain benign for years. Or it might have become the one domino that causes the entire structure to topple tomorrow. To treat a vulnerability you have to find its source—your weak link. Your weak link usually starts at the feet. Not that your weak link *is in* your feet, but your feet are the springboards to balance. A problem with your feet or legs, for example, can give you a pain in the neck.

Lenny limped into my office on a cane, wearing a knee brace. He complained about constant pain in his left knee. I learned that Lenny was an insurance salesman and that he worked sitting down. He talked to people all day long while seated. When he talked, I noticed that Lenny had a peculiar habit. In what I thought was an attempt to appear emphatic, he would jut his head forward and tilt it to one side.

I treat knee patients like I do all patients, as whole body patients. So I didn't start at the knee; I started by balancing his entire body. I checked his gait for weakness or tightness, in order to spot asymmetries that might contribute to his knee pain. I saw that his head was positioned too far forward, he leaned back when he walked, and he locked (overstraightened) his knees with each step (also called knee hyperextension).

In addition to working on his knee, we strengthened his abdomen and gave his spine greater flexibility. Lenny progressed nicely, and the pain in his knee subsided. That's when I began to suspect that his knee problem was actually sciatic pain that stemmed from a back problem. I learned more about his peculiar habit, too. Lenny had a hearing problem. *That's* why his head protruded forward. His head was forward *all* the time, which caused him to lean back to counterbalance his body's tendency to fall forward as he stood or walked. Leaning back put abnormal stress on his hips, one of the anchor points of the sciatic nerve. The sciatic nerve travels to the knee. It may seem like a circuitous trail, but the pain in his knee was likely caused by a weak link at the top: the forward position of his head.

Nerves branch off from the spinal cord and travel to specific parts of the body to innervate them (make them work). Those nerves carry different messages, such as the ones indicating hot, cold, pain, skin sensations, *and movement*. When a nerve is compressed or compromised, any muscle, tendon, or other structural part along that nerve's path can receive that message in the form of tingling, numbness, or pain.

Another patient of mine, Terry, was an electrical engineer in his early forties. He was married and had three kids and a basset hound named Boone. His family represented the best of Donna Reed and the Brady Bunch, except for Boone, who harbored a delirious, jet-lagged disposition. Terry had never sustained an injury in his life, except for a broken foot as a kid, suffered when his older brother catapulted him from the front porch onto the lawn using a contraption made of an old hammock and some bungee cords.

One Saturday afternoon, Terry had finished mowing the lawn and was reeling in the extension cord. The cord pulled taut. Boone had fallen asleep on it. Terry gave it a slight tug. Nothing. He whipped the cord softly. Boone moaned and snapped shut a yawn. Terry looked down at the lug. It definitely needed a scratch behind the ear, and then it needed to be nudged over so Terry could get to the cord. Terry leaned over, scratched Boone, and then attempted to lift him off the cord. *Whap!* His back shot into spasms of pain like he'd never felt before. He winced, dropped to the ground, and rolled over onto his back. The pain subsided. But when he tried to get up, the pain shot through the right side of his lower back. Terry fell to the ground again and winced. Boone licked Terry's ear.

All right, I made up that last part about Boone licking Terry's ear. Boone actually never moved. But the important thing is that Terry hurt his back while bending over to move his dog. By itself that motion could not have led to his injury without a preexisting weakness. When Terry finally made it in to my clinic three weeks after the Boone incident, the pain had subsided but had not gone away. The sharp pain in his back recurred at varying times, usually as the result of sitting at his desk for more than fifteen minutes or when he pushed or pulled something, even light objects like the vacuum cleaner. Sometimes it hurt when he was just standing around talking, and his first step out of bed each day was excruciating.

So I began the process of tracing his weak link, first by asking him questions about his physical condition and background (we'll provide you with those questions later in this book), and then by watching him walk (we'll also equip you with the tools you need to analyze your own PMP). Remember that Terry had had a broken ankle when he was a kid. And like most kids, he whined to have the cast removed. His leg itched. And the signatures and drawings had not only lost their novelty, they had coalesced into a dirty gravy-brown blur much akin to the inside of a burrito. Even his mother was anxious to have the cast removed. Off it went a week early.

Terry had some pain in his foot for several months after the cast was removed. Not much, but enough to make him take a short step on the right, so he became a left-sided walker. The left leg did the work and the right leg was just carried along. This was so subtle that no one noticed. As a result, his entire body subtly shifted to the left without his noticing it, either. As he grew up, all of his physical exercises and his work habits (he's an electrical engineer, so he sits at a computer most of the day) continued to magnify the shift. Because he was only a moderate weekend athlete, the muscles in his back and belly grew weak, and by the day of the Boone attack, weakness around his lower back had become so pronounced that he displaced a vertebra and ruptured a disk.

The spine consists of a stack of small bones, called vertebrae, which you can think of as all strung together like beads on a string. They're all supposed to be level, and on top of each other, with just enough gradations forward and backward to create our natural curves.

Nerve roots branch off from the spinal cord at each vertebral level. In between the vertebrae are little cushions called disks. Nerve roots are protected by these disks and vertebrae. The disks maintain space between the vertebrae to enable circulation into the nerves. If a disk is herniated, slipped, or ruptured, that can narrow the space and compress a nerve, which can send a message to your arms and legs in the form of pain.

> The spine is made up of twenty-four vertebrae (7 cervical, 12 thoracic, 5 lumbar), plus five more that constitute the sacrum, plus four more that constitute the coccyx (or tailbone). (A disk located between the sixth and seventh cervical vertebrae is thus labeled the C6, 7 disk.) The single most important job of the vertebral column is to protect the spinal cord, which runs down the center of the spine. The spinal cord and the nerve roots that occur at each vertebral level are made of nerve tissue. This fragile nerve tissue splits off from the spinal cord and goes to the arms, legs, and organs. When nerve tissue is pinched or compressed, it transmits pain or numbness. The sciatic nerve is the most common example. It runs down the spine and through the back of the legs. Most people think sciatica is a dire and complicated condition, but it simply can be an indication that the sciatic nerve is being compromised and needs more breathing room anywhere along its path.

Terry had a herniated disk and a concomitant squished nerve. His path to wellness began with a trip to his internist. The internist prescribed muscle relaxants and anti-inflammatories for the pain, which helped him during the day. But each morning his first step out of bed was still very painful. Since the medicine didn't provide anything close to the improvement he'd hoped for, his internist sent him to an orthopedic surgeon. His orthopedic surgeon gave Terry spinal injections called epidural blocks that prohibit the transmission of pain. These helped for a month or so, but ultimately the pain returned. The more pain he experienced, the more he shifted to the left and leaned back, which further compressed the nerve and aggravated the pain.

Terry finally turned to more alternative types of help, including two chiropractors and an acupuncturist, each of whom produced some positive results and measurable relief. But the pain kept coming back. He finally decided to go to the stratagem of last resort, surgery. But before they had the opportunity to tinker with him, a friend of his just happened to mention my success with the friend's back problems. Terry came in convinced that I was his final line of nonintrusive defense.

In our first session we began to balance his gait, shift his body back to the right, stabilize his lower back and belly, and strengthen his vertical superstructure through the sandwich system, which I'll describe in detail later. The results were immediate. Some would say miraculous. I wouldn't. His own mind and body constituted the miracle at work here. Terry experienced less pain in increments of about 20 percent with each session, so by the end of five sessions he was better balanced than he was before the violent attack by mad dog Boone.

The injuries I see are most frequently due to a preexisting condition (a weak link) that the victim is most often not even aware of. If three different people, each of the same approximate age, height, and weight, walk down a warehouse aisle and slip on a puddle of spilled beet juice, even though each walks at the same velocity, wears the same type of shoes, and slips at the same angle, the accident will likely produce three completely different injuries (or lack thereof). A person with a weak belly who tends to lean back might tend to blow out a lumbar disk. A person with shoulders that roll forward might tear a rotator cuff (a rotator cuff is like a sleeve of tendons that surround the shoulder joint). A person with a well-balanced body might not incur any serious injury at all and be back at work the next day. Anyway, the point is that over 85 percent of the patients I see incur their injuries from a source other than the one they cite to me. And it's my job, as a seasoned body detective, to find their weak links.

When patients enter my office, I watch them walk. I observe how they sit as they fill out their paperwork. No, I don't have two-way mirrors, and you won't see me peering around corners. I just watch. Unconscious movements indicate far more than words. I observe what's weak, what's tight, and which side is stronger. I notice if all the components are participating effectively or if a few are doing most of the work.

I watch for clues about their dispositions. Can you tell the difference between a shy person and an aggressive person at first glance? These characteristics influence how people hold themselves. People with low self-esteem often slump. People who are proud often strut with their heads high, frequently too high. The muscles and ligaments that support these poses trickle through the body and are reflected in a person's Primary Movement Pattern.

To strengthen *your* weak link, first I establish how you created it. By the time we get to my treatment room, I can usually guess what hurts. This book will show you how to sleuth it out on your own—and fix it.

How You Created Your Weak Link

Terry developed a weak link in his back that could be traced to a childhood foot injury. But there are many other ways in which people arrive at their own particular PMPs. Your PMP has fundamental roots starting with your genetic makeup. A hereditary predisposition to a round upper back, for example, could cause a walk characterized by a forward shoulder roll. When shoulders are rolled forward all the time, the muscles and ligaments around those joints take on the new position. They slowly adapt as they shorten on the front side and lengthen on the back side, a condition that becomes fixed or permanent *until treated*.

These adaptations are a cover-up that arise from the human body's attempt to correct itself. But they represent a nightmare for the physical therapist who's trying to sort it all out. Some adaptations cause new stresses elsewhere in the body. The body then becomes naturally used to being out of balance. Most people tell me they were "born that way" and "you can't change it." On the contrary, my experience shows that you walked into your current situation, and you can walk your way out of it as well.

For the majority of people, genetic predisposition plays a minor role compared to the following factors: (1) your developmental environment—how you learned to walk growing up, who you fashioned yourself after; (2) the things you do habitually, ritually, or otherwise repetitiously, including everything from how and where you work to how you blow-dry your hair or perform other daily chores; (3) injuries and illnesses from birth to the present, as with Terry and his wonder-dog Boone; and (4) exercise history, including the sports you play.

Developmental Environment

Gina, an advertising account executive, developed a peculiar hitch to her gait because of a childhood injury. In her early teens she'd fractured her clavicle (the bone that goes from your throat to your shoulder). To compensate for the pain, she developed a shoulder thrust that accompanied each step she took. As she stepped forward with her left foot, her right shoulder swung forward, followed by her arm and hand. Had she snapped her fingers with her right hand when she walked she would have looked like one of the Jets from *West Side Story*. She also had other quirks to her walk. But this case history isn't about Gina. It's about her seven-year-old daughter, Jesse.

I treated Gina for several months. Her PMP was on the upswing. She improved the hitch, regained her posture, and had completely eliminated her shoulder blade pain. It was a Wednesday afternoon, and Gina generally arrived on time. But on that particular day she was late. And, unlike her previous visits, this time she brought along her daughter, Jesse.

Here's the intriguing part. When Gina first walked into my office, she was followed by Jesse, who swung her right arm forward just like her mom. Jesse walked with the same hand swing and shoulder throw that Gina had prior to therapy. A little mini-Jet! Like most of us, when Jesse learned to walk, she emulated her mother.

The trillions of neurons in a child's brain wait to be programmed. Neurons from the retina connect to the brain's visual cortex with the first gathered information about sight. Neurons from parts of the body connect to neurons in the sensory-motor cortex about movement. At walking age, little children are virtual vacuum cleaners for data. By age ten, the circuits in the brain that regulate motor development have been finalized, making emulation an even stronger element in the child's learning process. How you walk is influenced by what you saw and who you emulated. Jesse clearly had an affinity for her mom's cool walk. Fortunately they both learned to balance their bodies and equalize their arm swing (Mom first, and then Jesse; both needed retraining).

Habits, Rituals, and Repetitive Motions

Anything you do repetitively has an impact on your Primary Movement Pattern, including, but to a lesser extent, nonambulatory activities such as sitting or doing dishes. Any activity that's constant in your life will influence your PMP. These habitual motions frequently slip by unnoticed. By the time they're discerned, the problem may already exist. Be aware of your own patterns as you read through this section.

Even physical therapists need physical therapy. Alice was a physical therapist with a perplexing problem: she couldn't identify her own source of misalignment. She came to me for help. Alice had developed a pervasive pain in her neck and shoulder, and it had progressed to the point that it was distracting her from her work.

Since she hadn't been able to diagnose her own ailment, she went to several outside experts. Her doctor identified a herniated C6, 7 disk. Shunning surgery, she tried a chiropractor. Then she tried acupuncture. She still had that burning pain in her neck and right shoulder. She came into my office because she'd heard about this PMP work of mine.

In our first three sessions, very little progress took place either in identifying her primary weak link or in reducing her pain. She leaned back slightly and held her head forward, and when we'd focus on that she'd feel better. But when she returned for her next session, she'd say that by the evening of her last session she'd had the same pain again.

By the end of her fourth visit I was genuinely frustrated by her ephemeral progress. After the session, I walked her halfway to the door and watched her as she gathered her things. I watched her walk. I watched her movement pattern—again. She approached the door. Her stride was near perfect. She slung the strap of her purse over her shoulder and opened the door. A big purse. On her right shoulder. "Wait!" I chirped. She turned. My grin was as big as a bathtub. I marched over and lifted her purse up by the strap. It weighed more than a weekend watermelon. I took her bag and crossed the strap over her head so the bag still hung on her right side but the strap hung off her left shoulder. We stared at each other as if we were two sisters who'd just met again for the first time in years. Sure enough, the problem was solved and she required no more physical therapy from me. She had to finish strengthening her shoulder, and she had to stretch and balance her body, but she could do those things on her own. Sometimes the obvious becomes apparent in its own sweet time.

Injuries and Illnesses

Terry's broken foot is a good example of how an injury can influence your Primary Movement Pattern. But nonbroken parts can be just as influential.

Jody was thirty-six, and a mother of three small children. She had been an "A" tennis player years before, but the kids came first now. Just recently she had undergone abdominal surgery and had been forced to stay in bed for six weeks. When she was finally up and around again, catching up on her graphic design business and dealing with the kids full-time prevented her from exercising at all.

Jody was an instinctive athlete rather than a biomechanically sound athlete. This meant that several structural vulnerabilities in her body were sitting ducks. The amount of time she'd spent in bed, and sitting at a computer all day, left her body weakened and deconditioned to the point that it was just a matter of which major joint was going to blow out first. It turned out to be her neck. She had a beautiful, long neck, and although she was very graceful, she leaned back when she walked and her head was overly forward. This compounded her vulnerability.

One day while she was in the middle of a business conversation on her cordless phone, she walked by the kitchen door and noticed her youngest child constructing a food mosaic on the kitchen counter. The composition was made of Cheerios, cheese puffs, and sauerkraut, all beautifully offset with contrasting sunset hues of peach yogurt. The shock of the discovery wasn't as disturbing as the fact that the artist was in the process of knocking over a jar of strawberry jam, which Jody lunged to catch but could not. A second mosaic was in progress on the terra-cotta floor, and Jody's diving miss gave her a shocking pain through the right side of her neck.

Her doctor sent her to me for cervical traction, but a quick look at her gait revealed a very pronated right foot and an obviously weak right sartorius muscle (her knee rolled in and locked with every step). Jody's right hip was weak, and her body dropped to the right with each step of her right foot. She held her head slightly to the right because her neck pain was on the right side.

Correcting her gait from the floor up did wonders. Strengthening came easily for her because she was an athlete and knew how to take directions. With time, she got back on track with a new gait that, along with appropriate exercises, gave her the strength she'd lost as a result of her illness, bed rest, children, and her job.

Exercise History

Another significant factor in determining your PMP is exercise history. If your background included formal ballet, for example, the hip turnout could cause you to lean back. This could lead to hip problems, since more than likely your hips would be your weakest link. This isn't to say that it's bad to dance ballet with extreme hip turnout—unless you can't turn back in and walk normally, like Devorah. She was fifty years old. She was also a ballet instructor. She'd been dancing since she was ten and had arabesqued her way around the world.

Devorah limped into my office one day looking way too haggard for an otherwise healthy, light, bright, well-exercised, limber woman. She complained that her right hip was on fire and her entire right leg hurt. Before she said a word I'd noticed that she had so much "toe turnout" that from the waist down she looked like Goofy, but with much smaller feet. She simply couldn't stand with her toes pointing straight ahead unless she applied tremendous strain. The attempt alone caused agonizing pain in her right hip.

Internal hip rotator muscles are used to turn the hips in, which is the motion you make as you point your big toes toward each other. External hip rotator muscles are the ones you use to point the toes out like duck feet (for example, Goofy and Devorah). Devorah had overused her external rotators and weakened her internal rotators to the point of atrophy.

By overusing her external rotators, her piriformis muscle was too tight, which put pressure on the sciatic nerve. This pressure intensified because she walked leaning back. This common malady is called Piriformis Syndrome. Unfortunately, this syndrome is commonly misdiagnosed as a disk disorder because both produce sciatic pain.

Sciatic pain, which often connotes wildly feared images of the worst kind of pain, is merely a description of any discomfort that's caused by impingement of the sciatic nerve, either at the nerve root (as in the case of a ruptured disk) or anywhere along the nerve's pathway. It's common for this type of nerve compression to occur just under the piriformis muscle when your feet turn out or you lean back a lot. That's because the sciatic nerve runs just under the piriformis muscle. So when the muscle tightens too much it squeezes down on the nerve. Disk problems are not necessarily the cause of sciatic pain.

It took months of stretching to get Devorah's feet back in so her toes faced straight ahead and to strengthen her internal hip rotators. To balance the hip joints, both the internal and external hip rotators must be strong. She began to balance her body and decompress her lower back, taking pressure off her right hip. She will always have to nurse her hip along by strengthening and stretching, but her newly balanced body will keep her cleanly distanced from severe pain.

One might question why her right hip hurt and not her left, or both hips. The answer is that no one is perfectly symmetrical. Each of us has a side that's stronger and more flexible than the other, which can be traced to any one or a combination of the elements described in this chapter. I'm a left-sided walker, though a subtle version. Devorah was a right-sided walker, an extreme version. She powered her gait with her right side, which fatigued first.

The piriformis muscle, located deep in the buttock muscle, crosses from the tailbone to the outer hip joint. This muscle was constantly tightened, putting abnormal pressure on her lumbar nerve. This compressed her sciatic nerve, which is part of the lumbar plexus, which runs just under the piriformis muscle and down into the leg, which caused her leg pain. (See piriformis muscle in Appendix B on page 269.)

PROBLEM POSTURE ABSOLUTELY
LEADS TO PAIN

After years of observation, and having treated a multitude of patients, I have narrowed down the four most common posture-related problems. Because of the way the human body has evolved, the back is the most structurally vulnerable part, at least as it's influenced by posture. If you look at a side view of a human skeleton, you can see how the whole top half of the body, the heavier half, is supported by the pelvis. That's why leaning back, or "sitting in your hips," creates more pressure on the lower back than it was intended to endure and why it causes problems. Leaning back is so common, at one point I thought of titling this book *Don't Lean Back.*

The gait of a runway model is the perfect example of how to walk with structural *im*balance. Picture a model walking down a long runway. Each step is straight down the middle, and her feet actually cross her midline. That narrow base of support can lead to problems because it causes her to lean back. Anything less wide than your hips constitutes a narrow base of support and elicits leaning back. The muscles located in your sides are summoned to balance the body, creating a slight side-to-side waddle. The muscles that should be stabilizing your spine, the ones at your abdomen and lower back, aren't used much. Disuse makes them weak, which causes more leaning back.

Now picture the model as she turns at the end of the runway. She stops, turns, and coquettishly fiddles with her little coat. Her shoulders are back. At this point, most of her entire body weight is in her hips. She's leaning so far back that her hips even appear to be thrust forward. Because she's ultra-lean, very young, and carrying no extra weight other than the clothes she's wearing, she's able to continue this repeatedly without major pain . . . so far.

Leaning back is by far the most common PMP deviation. About nine out of ten people with problematic posture tend to lean back, shifting their center of gravity from in front of the main support

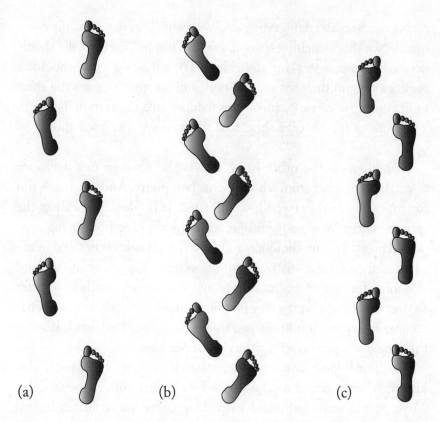

1-1 (a) Correct: feet turned out at fifteen to twenty degrees (b) Incorrect: feet turned out too far (c) Incorrect: no turnout at all

(hips, legs, and feet) to behind the main support (hip sitting). The trunk relaxes and rests in the hip joints. To counterbalance this stance or gait, the natural inclination is to roll the shoulders, neck, and head forward to keep from falling backward. If I had a dollar for every time I've told a patient to stop leaning back, I would only have a couple of thousand dollars. But if I had just one penny for every hip sitter on the planet, I could toast every sunset with a celebratory Bordeaux and buy a palatial château in southern France in which to drink it.

The second most common deviation is raising the rib cage upward and out. "Pull your shoulders back," a command barked out by both caring mothers and denigrating drill sergeants, was not a healthy command. Not that slouching is good. It's not. But pulling back the shoulders overcompensates for slouching. Try thrusting your shoulders back, away from their natural position, and see how it causes the chest to lift up. That creates structural instability (see illustration 1-2, [c]). The front of the rib cage should be tilted down. The back should be up.

Slouching, on the other hand, causes the rib cage to tilt too far down, making your stomach stick out. Not pretty. And not much fun for your spine, either (see illustration 1-2, [b]). Slouching causes the spine to curve incorrectly and prevents the rib cage from being supported properly. The shoulders roll forward in an attempt to counterbalance the uneven distribution of weight. Try standing up and slouching for just a minute. Notice that your weight tends to transfer to your heels and that it's easy for your shoulders to roll forward. That compensatory motion keeps you from falling over backward. It's also the stance of a person who sits in his or her hips.

The third most common deviation is locking the knees, also known as hyperextending the knees. That's when they're too straight. Most people walk and stand with their knees forced into a locked position. Some even push them back so far that they appear to curve backward. Locking the knees comes naturally to most people as a means of providing a firm base of support. But it's altogether inefficient. After years of relying on locked knees to support the body, the muscles that you could have been using become flaccid and weak. Pretty soon it seems like you can't stand still without locking your knees. Although this chapter is devoted to how you walked into pain, not how to walk away from it, the correct leg position is very slightly bent, or just unlocked.

The last of the common deviations occurs when your ankles roll in toward each other. This is called having pronated feet—a.k.a., flat feet. Although flat feet might be something you think you were born with, this deviation can be improved or sometimes corrected by changing the way you walk. The muscles surrounding the ankles, and some of your hip muscles, just need strengthening. And since your

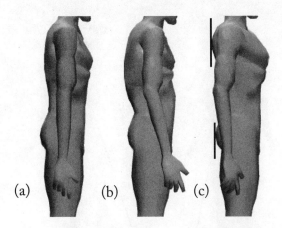

(a)   (b)   (c)

1–2 (a) Correct: ribcage and shoulders in correct position, spinal curve normal (b) Incorrect: shoulders forward with ribs down and forward, spinal curve lost (c) Incorrect: rib cage raised up and out. Note how shoulders are behind buns, which is not correct.

feet are handling the majority of the load, it behooves you to train the feet to carry it.

When the feet roll in, your knees tend to lock, which forces the weight of the torso to sit in the hips, resulting in the infamous leaning back position. The shoulders, neck, and head move forward in an effort to compensate for the backward shift. This posture changes your center of gravity and puts tremendous stress on your lower back and neck.

A healthy back position is one in which the body's weight is evenly distributed throughout the entire spine. Postural deviations, such as leaning back, create stress at the joints between vertebrae, particularly in the lumbar region and in the neck, which are the primary pivotal points and the two major apexes of the spine's curve. When jeopardized in any way, or when out of balance, back muscles tense up into protective reflexive positions and become virtual splints that hold the joint still. This means they don't move naturally, and they grow weaker, leading to vulnerability and eventually to an injury. This chain of imbalance makes something as innocuous as bending over to scratch your dog turn into a mass of perpetual pain.

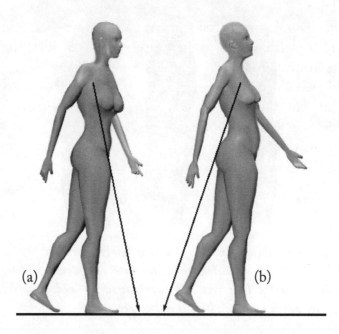

1–3 (a) Correct walking posture, with center of gravity forward (b) Incorrect walking posture, with center of gravity to the back

Common deviations lead to pain, and that pain might pop up anywhere in your body. Pronated feet might explain the pain in your hip. Correcting pronated feet can solve backaches and neck aches. The chain reactions that cause soreness in some distant parts of the body are usually caused by some fundamental imbalance elsewhere, often starting in the feet.

People used to think that we were born with behavior patterns, or that they were something that just happened to us. Freud dissuaded us from that misconception decades ago. We learn behavior, we don't inherit it. Your Primary Movement Pattern was learned. You might have learned it so deeply that it seems locked in forever, and trying to change it may feel completely unnatural. The eye-opening truth is that what feels familiar may be exactly what's causing your pain.

Sometimes it takes a near-tragic experience—like the death of a loved one, divorce, or a debilitating injury—for a person to finally grasp the significance of an unsuccessful pattern that's been repeated over and over. It's human nature to lack motivation until that traumatic event hits. Fear and pain are great motivators, but they don't have to precede change. And fortunately, you have the capacity to change all the time. You're in the cockpit. All you need is the desire to arrive safely at your destination. This book contains the flight plan. But first, maybe you'll want to pour that cup of tea and think a little about how you might have walked your way into pain.

≋ 2 ≋

YOU CAN WALK
YOURSELF WELL
EVERYONE CAN DO IT AND YOU CAN, TOO

THE HANDS-OFF APPROACH

For the first few years of my private practice, I thought that developing my hands would make me a healer. I took courses on all kinds of massage, acupressure, joint mobilization, stretch facilitation techniques, and just about anything that looked like it might have therapeutic benefit. My practice grew as my hands became more skillful. But there was something missing in all these "hands-on" methods. They all created results, but there were inherent short-term limitations, and my patients were always coming back for further treatment. Flattered as I was, I knew there was something very wrong.

Physical therapists, like other doctors and medical practitioners, are expected to fix patients like auto mechanics repair cars. Patients expect modalities such as ultrasound, or electric stimulation, or maybe even masterful healing hands to anoint and massage their pain away. When people misunderstand how their own bodies work, they want to assign responsibility for their well-being to someone else. They want to be fixed by having things done to them: "My knee hurts. Fix my knee." The result is that patients give us their power.

That's not what we're up to here. This book is about you fixing yourself. It's sort of like the old adage about the starving family. Give them bread, feed them for a day. Give them seed and a hoe, feed them for a lifetime. This is not magic; it's science. But I can tell you emphatically that there is something at work here that is powerful, comprehensive, and cosmic. It's your mind. The road to healing requires its full participation.

As was noted previously, structural pain is caused by a weak link in the body, often not where you experience pain. Nerves are like road maps. They run all over the place, so that a pinched nerve in your lower spine, for example, might cause pain in your leg. That's why it's important to treat the body as a complete entity. It ensures that the true source of the pain isn't overlooked in a mad dash for a quick fix. Comprehensive, durable healing is usually more than an isolated repair. One of the saddest stories I hear, yet one that comes up over and over again, is about a surgery that not only didn't remove the pain but has now caused the patient lost time and new complications.

A patient of mine named Miranda was living off her credit cards, and yet she was terrified to go back to work. She was afraid her body wouldn't hold up after her second surgery had failed. Her first was a bomb, so she'd gone to another orthopedic surgeon out of desperation. After her second orthopedic surgery failed, and all the drugs, injections, and bed rest didn't resolve her pain, she was in a near panic. She explained her situation to her internist, who sent her to me. I often get the human version of stray kittens, and I don't mind a bit when they've got a positive attitude like hers.

Miranda turned out to be one of the most diligent patients I've ever encountered. She was a fantastic listener. She was joyful about the various corrections and exercises I showed her, and her attitude about recovery was exemplary. I remember the day she broke through for good. She tearfully told me, as she glided gracefully back and forth in my gym, "I feel like I'm back in control of my own body." She looked like she was walking on air with her new gait. Here was a woman with the personal power to treat herself (though lacking the knowledge at the time), who in good conscience elected to entrust a team of surgeons first. Knowledge, combined with belief in one's self, can lead to a much safer and stabler form of healing.

PAIN AS A CRUTCH

Remember the story about Stephanie from the introduction? She was the thirty-eight-year-old sound engineer who smashed up her VW and developed shoulder pain that remained even after her crash wounds healed. Stephanie recovered completely, but it took more time than it should have. Here's why.

When Stephanie crashed her VW, she had been drinking. Actually, she was quite drunk. She smashed into, among other things, a nice old lady complete with grandma status. Besides suffering a broken arm and developing a few more gray hairs, she was okay. But Stephanie didn't handle the guilt too well. She was emotionally devastated, consumed with self-derision, which gave her a compelling reason not to recover. She didn't believe she deserved it.

When a person feels he or she deserves pain, or that he or she is weak, incapable, or powerless, these mental barriers make physical recovery extremely challenging. In Stephanie's case, there was a bonus booby prize that worked against her recovery—her husband adored taking care of her, so there was a built-in payoff for continued pain.

Growing up in my house, we got so much love and attention when we were sick that it actually became fun. Comic books, Popsicles, Jell-O, and Mom at home, all day. One of my old tricks was to get sick to increase intimacy with my mother. This tendency, common among young children, is sometimes carried over into adulthood. Finding the good in a negative situation is commendable, but using pain as a tool is not.

As you sit down with that cup of tea to think about how you might have walked into pain, think about all the reasons you want to improve yourself, eliminate pain, and get on with your life. You must know that you deserve good health, and you must not have any subconscious motivations that might reward, slow, or impair recovery.

LETTING GO

These situations are not the only ones that hamper the normal recovery process. More often, what gets in the way is resistance to the concept of changing something so seemingly permanent and entrenched—the way you walk.

People arrive at my office with all kinds of attitudes and preconceived expectations. Despite what they come in with, they eventually experience their first magical moment of success, and that electrifies and motivates both of us. I can count on it as surely as the sun rises, from the flaccid to the brittle, from the unathletic to the Olympic contender, young, old, confident, shy, large, tiny, and so on. They all get there. It goes something like this:

During our first session, I can see my patients looking at me, trying not to let their eyes pop out, hoping I won't see their own skepticism regarding their ability to change. They think they're too old, or too uncoordinated, or just too untrainable to change their walk. They say, "Me? Oh no, I just can't."

Many people think that changing the way they walk is like parting the Red Sea. Even the notion of changing the way they walk sounds painfully ridiculous and clumsy. Then I point to the Japanese symbol on my wall. The symbol stands for the word *chaos*, which carries with it the following Zen meaning: "Before the beginning of great brilliance, there must be chaos. Before a brilliant person begins something great, they must look foolish to the crowd."

The beauty of this concept is that if my patients give themselves permission to look ridiculous and get it wrong, it's shortly thereafter that they begin to get it right.

• • •

A highly driven businessman named James came into my office with what I could sense was a skeptical attitude. He was one of those patients who thought that changing the way he walked was like being brainwashed. In addition to his skepticism, James was angry, too. Angry with his body. Angry at his pain. Angry that I didn't fix him with some kind of magic wand.

I showed him how to correct his own back pain, starting with his gait. James listened to my words and watched my demonstrations, but without concentration. He'd pay attention for a bit, but as soon as I attempted to change the way he walked, he'd go into mental hibernation.

The next time I saw James, he had excuses for why he couldn't practice, or exercise, and why he didn't appear to have made any progress. The next week the same thing happened. I sat down with James, looked him in the eyes, and asked him what was really going on. He confessed. He said he found it hard to believe that changing the way he walked would reduce his pain.

I took a deep breath and softened. I looked away. Scanning my mind for the speech I knew so well, I turned back to James. I told him it was okay that he was skeptical. I explained that the strengthening exercises alone would help a lot and that since he had to walk anyway, he might as well try the corrections just in case they helped. I asked him to give it two weeks and if there was no improvement, we'd regroup. James promised to practice and do his exercises. When he came back the next week, he was all smiles. He said he was experiencing less than half the pain. He felt relieved, and he radiated satisfaction.

Most of my patients go through the analysis phase relatively painlessly. Then I introduce some corresponding corrective measures. When we get to the part where they walk, people say all kinds of funny things. Some say "I feel like Groucho Marx," and they crouch down and pretend to smoke cigars. Some say "I feel like a gorilla," and they scratch somewhere. Some women say the corrected walk is too manly or too assertive. Some men say it's too swishy or too bouncy. Some guys even suffer remorse over having to give up their cool strut!

These are emotional reactions that arise as patients come face-to-face with change. The ones who have the hardest time are those who are afraid of another failed attempt at removing their pain. Others worry about how they will appear to others with their new walks. (This "new walk," incidentally, eventually looks as vibrant and attractive as it is structurally sound.)

Changing your Primary Movement Pattern will feel awkward and unnatural at first. But the gait that feels natural is almost invariably your comfort zone gait. Your old gait is the one that's causing the problems in the first place. Once you open up to that possibility, adapting to change becomes much easier.

Now, back to that first magical moment of success I referred to at the start of this section. After a session or two, it happens. They let go, almost accidentally, of all that self-conscious stuff that they've been blushing about. They suddenly recognize that they've experienced a perceptible sense of lightness. Gravity seems less powerful. Their bodies are balanced for the first time in their lives, and they can feel it. The light goes on, their faces soften, and then I get comments like "Maybe I'm dreaming that this takes the pressure off my spine" and "I swear, this does feel better." A few weeks later, they respond with comments like "Can you show me how I used to walk? I can't remember what it looked like!" I show them, and they laugh. I'm moved, knowing that what I've shown them is no more than a simple path to structural common sense that will last them a lifetime.

Gravity does not have to dictate your posture or cause you to surrender to movement patterns by default. Once you start to feel balanced, and your muscles do the work that used to be distributed to your joints, you too will experience a sense of lightness, an uplifting feeling. You may not be sure why, but you'll feel better. That experience will inspire you onward. You won't think you're dabbling away at some rote, disciplinary exercises that miss the big picture. You'll feel stronger. And you'll carry that stature with you everywhere you go for the rest of your life. Leona was seventy-seven years old when she came to me. This was her second visit. As the result of a hip replacement, her right leg was a bit shorter than her left. The wide left step I asked her to try wasn't so bad, at least not with the help of her cane, but when I brought her weight forward and talked about changing the way she walked, again, I could see the same resistance I'd seen with James.

She looked at me like I'd just told her to sing "Mac the Knife" in Portuguese. The look continued as if to say that she would patiently fake her way through whatever torture I threw at her, but as soon as she got outside, she was going to toddle about with her same old deviated gait.

I asked her what her motivation was for coming to see me. Oh, sure, I knew she wanted to remove pain and get around with greater ease. But I wanted to know what she really wanted beyond mobility. She said she really wanted to get back into golf. Just a few holes of par 3 would satisfy her. I told her if she diligently practiced what I was about to show her, not much would prevent her from shooting eighteen holes soon.

Leona's eyes got wide. She stared at me as if to say, "Hand me that accordion, stand back, and how do you say 'When that shark bites' in Portuguese?" Changing something that's been habitual for decades is not simple, but once you make the mental shift, you're well on the way to structural balance.

SELF-GUIDED LEARNING

Once you have read, learned, and practiced what's in this book, that's it. There is no attaining a higher level with respect to the way you walk. You will be balanced, and as long as you don't relearn old habits, you'll stay that way.

To learn your new way of walking, we've provided a series of evaluative questions that lead you to your own specific gait corrections. Each correction is offered in an easy-to-follow, step-by-step fashion. Work on three corrections at a time—or more, if you are so inclined. Along with most gait corrections come some corresponding exercises. They are not complicated, and you absolutely *can* do them.

The most effective approach is to take four walks a day focusing on your new movement pattern. Each walk can be just five minutes long, and they should be spread out during the day. As you practice, you'll also find it helps to verbalize the corrective processes to reinforce your assimilation of the techniques. You will be encouraged to repeat the verbal part to yourself like a mantra: "Up and over, breathe sideways, unlock your knees, and widen your stance."

It will feel unnatural at first, but it's easy. All it takes is five minutes, four times a day.

I remember an ob-gyn named David who used to call me from the locker room floor of his hospital. He'd be stuck there, lying on his back, trying to untangle himself from another series of back spasms. These usually hit him after a late-night delivery. The fourth time he called me from the floor I told him we couldn't go on meeting like this, and that he would have to start doing his exercises and practice. He said, "What makes you think I haven't been?" I asked him what the view was like from the floor, and if he really enjoyed it more than his exercises.

In the beginning, David said he didn't have time for the exercises. But that night, when I helped him on-site for the fourth time, he explained that he couldn't see how the exercises were going to help, and he wasn't even sure if he was doing them correctly when he did them. Since he was a doctor, I hesitated to go into the same simple explanations that I give my other patients as to why we were doing what we were doing. I thought he might feel that I was talking down to him and that we shared an unspoken insight into the human body that preempted exercise explanations. But I learned that he, too, needed to have that connection explained.

Every gait correction and exercise in this book comes with a detailed explanation of *why* you're doing it. Nothing is rote. Everything has a purpose that you need to understand in order to know if you're doing it correctly. When you understand how your body works, the process of reclaiming your personal power also expands.

At first, your movements will be a conscious effort. But eventually your new walk will become so natural that it won't require any mental effort at all. It will become your new unconscious style of walking.

Until then, your natural inclination will be to revert to your old style of movement. That's why you will need to learn to feel your muscles and consciously focus on relearning some simple motions.

Try bending your arm and putting your hand to your mouth. Feel the muscles that make this movement possible? Bring your hand to your mouth again, but this time put tension in your biceps muscle and tense your forearm and wrist. You can feel the muscles at work. You can add or subtract muscle tension with your brain. You are in charge of reprogramming your body with version 1.0 of your new gait!

BODY DETECTIVE AND HEALER

People get embarrassed when I ask them to feel their buns contract as they walk. Okay, so it's a little personal to talk about your buns and how they feel, but knowing at which point during your walk your bun muscles have contracted is relevant. When I ask patients if they know when their bun muscles tense up during their walk, they invariably say, "I have no idea." Soon you will know. You will learn to know what muscles are active during all stages of your walk. You'll be aware of movements that generate pain, too. You are going to play Sherlock Holmes with your body.

The worst case of leaning back I can remember was a patient of mine named Georgia. She had never used her buns, or so it appeared. Her rear end had virtually disappeared through lack of use, which made her pants real baggy back there because there was nothing to fill them. Making things more odd, she looked pregnant but wasn't. She was fifty-five years old and a schoolteacher. Except for the middle of her, she was thin. And Georgia was extremely bright. She'd obviously lived her life in her brain, using her body as a carrying case that never received much attention.

You might have guessed that Georgia hated exercise. She lived on anti-inflammatories to help her back pain, but it worsened to the point that she was forced to respond to her body's demands. That's when she slumped into my office, clueless as to what it felt like to use the muscles in the middle of her. I asked her if she could feel her bun muscles when she walked, or ever. She blushed, looked down, and adjusted her glasses.

It took a long time, and some studious core strengthening, but now Georgia can tell you exactly when her buns are contracting. She took on the project of improving her body like it was a classroom subject. She looks gorgeous now, and she wouldn't give up her new gait, or her daily exercise and swimming, for anything.

It isn't easy to take responsibility for your own health and to see yourself as your own healer. Soon, however, you will hit that first magical moment of success and realize that you are in control. That will be an extremely empowering insight, after which you'll quickly allow your intuition to guide the way to new discoveries about your balancing mechanisms. You will become your own teacher, doctor, and therapist. When you finally let go of your doubts about whether you can know how your body works, you might make observations about the human body that I'm not even aware of. Some of my most rewarding experiences come when my patients explain their own discoveries, and *they're teaching me*.

All humans are driven to embrace growth. They may deny it, as they stubbornly muddle forward, but their subconscious drive to survive eventually takes command. Patients may come to me with all sorts of attitudes, but they're listening to me for a reason. They want to change. That's why they come in, and that's why you're reading this book. So it's vital that you understand the concepts presented in this book well enough to make the change and own it forever.

Taking charge of your health means more than going to the gym, or taking daily walks, or eating well. It includes understanding the dynamics of your body. It's a twenty-four-hour-a-day process. Spending an hour on yourself won't work if the other twenty-three are spent doing damage without knowing it.

I believe in my patients' abilities to survive and improve. My belief in them is usually more powerful than their bouts of recalcitrance, moodiness, defeatism, embarrassment, or lethargy. But in this case, my belief in your ability won't help you much. It's *your* belief that's vital.

3

HUMAN BALANCE AND MOTION

WHAT DOES A CORRECT WALK LOOK LIKE?

Because every body has different dimensions, proportions, and genetic coding, its hard to imagine a one-size-fits-all standard for symmetrical walking. The truth is that height, weight, proportions, age, sex, and all other human features and options don't change the basic elements of a symmetrical walk. When it comes to holding yourself up against the gravitational pull of the earth and propelling yourself forward, the biomechanics of human motion are consistent. Human symmetry has simple standards, and these standards apply to you.

To understand the interrelationship of all the elements that comprise a well-balanced Primary Movement Pattern (your walk) it's important to acknowledge that balance starts at the feet, the point at which you and the ground become contiguous. The rest of the balancing act, and how it involves all your other body parts, is only as good as your footing. With that obvious point in mind, it should come as no surprise that most imbalance begins, or manifests, at the feet, then trickles up in various compensations throughout the body all the way to your head.

BALANCE AND MOTION

Your body extends upward from your feet on stanchions. These stanchions, your legs, attach to the back of the feet, not the middle. It's important to visualize a perpendicular stick attached to the back of a horizontal block the way your leg attaches to your foot. Visualizing this connection should enable you to see that when the foot hits the ground improperly, the entire body loses its balance to the rear. Your rump isn't padded for nothing.

With legs at the rear of the feet, and the body's natural inclination to lose balance to the rear, the most common of all walking deviations is to lean back. That should seem harmless enough, but leaning back as you walk destroys your symmetry. Everything that comes naturally is not necessarily symmetrical or healthful. Some natural inclinations come from following the path of least resistance, from learned bad habits, or are copied from a parent.

Since the first thing to hit the ground in a footstep is the heel, it should make sense that a balanced step begins at the heel's center. Most people, however, will find that their heel strikes to the outside, or to the inside, more than in the center. This misalignment causes the foot to fight for balance any way it can, and most often leads to

3–1 (a) Inside heel strike (b) Neutral heel strike (c) Outside heel strike

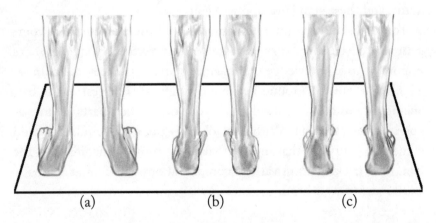

(a)   (b)   (c)

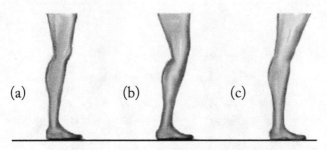

(a)   (b)   (c)

3–2 (a) Correct: knee soft, slightly forward (b) Incorrect: knee bent too far forward (c) Incorrect: knee hyperextended (bent back)

what's called pronation, or a rolling inward. Odd as it may seem, both misplaced heel strikes, whether to the inside or the outside, usually lead to foot pronation at some point during the step.

Pronated feet almost always force the knees into a locked position to break what would be a backward fall, which makes your top half balance like a teeter-totter on your bottom half. This in turn forces you to sit in your hips (rest your body's weight in your hip joints) in order to gain some semblance of balance. This is a bad connection between your two halves. It may be so subtle that you don't know you're doing it. You'll gain much more insight into this as you continue reading. A more genuine connection is made when your muscle strength, both abdomen and back, is sandwiching your body together upright against gravity, holding your torso erect without dumping the load onto your hip joints.

The common deviation of hip sitting throws the weight of the body backward. To compensate, the head and shoulders thrust forward in an effort to achieve some sort of balance. That little sequence is absolutely the most common series of events that leads to structural pain. Keep in mind that weakness and/or pain do not always pop up in the same place for everyone. *That's* where body type and proportions come in. Injuries invariably occur at a person's weak link.

At times, the sequence that results in imbalance is initiated at another part of the body. In chapter 1 you read about Lenny, who jutted his head way out because he was hard of hearing. His compen-

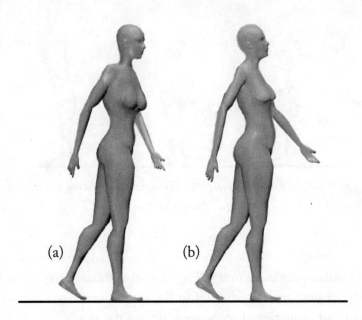

3–3 (a) Correct walking posture (b) Hip sitter with head and shoulders forward

satory mechanism went from top to bottom. It can really start anywhere on the body, but since the most common sequence is bottom to top, that's the direction I'll take as I describe the makeup of a well-balanced Primary Movement Pattern.

THE STANCE AND SWING PHASES OF WALKING

Every step we take has two phases: a stance phase and a swing phase. The stance phase is the part of walking when the foot is touching the ground. The three parts to the stance phase are: (1) *heel strike*, when only the heel is on the ground; (2) *mid-stance*, when the foot and toes come to the ground; and (3) *pushoff*, when the foot lifts onto the toes, which bend, squeeze down, and propel us forward, mostly with the big and middle toe.

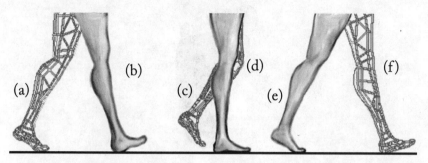

3–4 Stance phase (b) Heel strike (d) Mid-stance (e) Pushoff, and Swing phase (a) Pushoff (c) Swing (f) Heel strike

The swing phase is everything that happens between the time that the toes go airborne until the heel of the same foot strikes the ground again. Both stance and swing phases play a primary role in propelling us forward with optimal balance.

During the stance phase, there's a brief moment when the body's weight is entirely supported on one foot while the other foot is in its swing phase, moving through the air. Imagine an oddly shaped bag of bones balancing on a stick with a little foot on the end, all off to one side, and all moving forward. What a trick.

Now imagine how easy it is to do it imperfectly. If your heel strikes dead center and your weight passes evenly toward the outside of your foot during midstance, and your big and middle toes accomplish the pushoff, yippee! That's correct. A toddler gets it right immediately. For the ideal heel strike, take a look at a baby's footprint (see illustration 3–5). Later on we'll look at your heel strike to see if it's too far to the outside or the inside. If it is, it could be the culprit that's throwing your entire body out of balance.

During the swing phase, the leg bends and shortens so that it clears the ground as it moves forward. Since the leg that's moving forward is about the same length as the one it's about to pass, it makes sense that it shortens up a bit. Otherwise it might flail sideways to gain clearance, or even drag past the stance phase leg, and that's very low-tech. (How many of you remember being told to stop dragging your feet?) So the leg shortens by bending in three places:

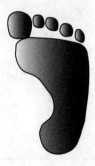

3–5 Baby's footprint—proper heel strike

the hip, the knee, and the ankle. During a proper swing phase, the primary muscle at work is the hip flexor, a powerful upper thigh muscle that bends the hip for foot clearance.

People who lean back when they walk develop their own special kind of compensatory mechanisms for getting their legs through the swing phase. They literally bounce their feet off the ground to shorten their swing leg instead of using their powerful hip flexor muscle. As a result, their hip flexor muscles grow weak through disuse, thus making them further dependent on the bounce method.

Other people who lean back use a mechanism called hip-hiking, in which they lift the entire hip to shorten their swing leg. This movement is accomplished by reducing the distance between the hip and the armpit, using the quadratus lumborum muscle, located above the hip. It actually goes from the top of the hip to the bottom of the lowest rib. (Try lifting your hip toward your rib and feel what it's like.) Once again, this leaves the hip flexors weak and the gait unoptimized.

Before describing the appearance of a proper stance, it's important to see what's happening during each of the two phases (stance and swing) from the floor up. Then you can really appreciate how all of the support stanchions and connectors—ankles, knees, hips, torso, neck, and head—have the capacity to contribute to symmetry and balance in motion. Keeping in mind that the stance phase is your balancing act on one foot, something else is going on that is equally bizarre. Not only is the entire weight of the body held up on one foot, but the body is actually twisting on itself as it moves forward. Imagine a toy doll for a minute and what she would look like if you held her shoulders and rotated them to the left while you held her hips and rotated them to the right. The momentum for the twist actually comes from the mid torso.

Now I'll describe the proper Primary Movement Pattern from the ground up, starting with the body parts used during the stance phase and then moving on to the swing phase.

The Stance Phase

In this section, we'll describe what each body part should be doing at each point of the stance phase—heel strike, mid-stance, and pushoff.

The Feet in the Stance Phase The feet in the stance phase are so vital that we've already covered the important issues earlier in this chapter. Here's a recap:

Heel strike: The feet should strike in the center of the heel.

Mid-stance: The body's weight should pass over the outside (not the outer edge, but near the outer edge) of the bottom of your foot.

Pushoff: The big and middle toes should push into the floor as if you're pulling the ground back, like on a treadmill.

The Ankles in the Stance Phase The ankle should be tight, not wobbly, and well supported from heel strike throughout pushoff. Ankle stability primarily comes from muscles located at the sides of the foot, from the lower leg, and, surprisingly, from the hips.

Heel strike: The ankle is flexed or bent. This is mostly accomplished by a muscle called the anterior tibialis. When this muscle isn't doing its job well, the strength needed to hold up the foot is compromised, often resulting in a malady referred to as "shin splints" (especially for runners).

Mid-stance: Muscles in the hip pull the knee open so that it faces slightly outward. That lifts the ankle so that it doesn't collapse into a flat, or pronated, foot

Pushoff: The heel should stay on the ground for as long as possible, lightly stretching the calf muscle and its Achilles tendon so the ankle is forced into flexion in preparation for pushoff.

> The muscle groups involved here are at the side of foot (peroneals), in the lower leg (extensor digitorum and tibialis anterior), and in the thigh (sartorius, the longest muscle in the human body). (See muscle illustrations in Appendix B on page 269.)

The Knees in the Stance Phase

Heel strike: The knee should be soft and spongy, not locked or rigid. The inside of the knee should feel like a big hard-boiled egg, so it can easily give with whatever texture the ground is.

Mid-stance: The knee is also loose at mid-stance, and the quads and hamstrings should be working hard to hold the knee firm and *nearly* straight.

Pushoff: The leg is slightly behind the body and the knee is very nearly straight, but still not locked back.

> The muscles involved here are mainly the quadriceps, which are your knee extensors, and the hamstrings, which are your knee flexors. (See Appendix B, page 269, for more information on flexors and extensors.)

The Hips in the Stance Phase

Heel strike: The hip flexors (muscles in the front of your hips that bend the trunk and legs toward each other) should be slightly bent and relaxed, having done their job already when they lifted the leg forward in the swing phase. The hip extensors (bun muscles) start to go into action by tightening to hold the upper body from falling forward.

Mid-stance: The hip is tight at the front. The back and outer hip muscles push inward so that the hip joint doesn't collapse too far to the outside and look like a Mae West pose.

Pushoff: The buns contract to create the length of the next step. They squeeze and lift the body slightly as it travels over the foot, balancing and stabilizing the lower torso with a firm foundation on which to swivel. Also at pushoff, the inner thigh contracts to create the width of the next step. You can feel your inner thigh muscles at work if you take unusually wide steps. These muscles power the leg to the width of the next step.

Try taking a few long, wide steps to feel your bun muscles contract—if your steps are wide enough you should be able to feel your inner thigh muscles, too.

> The muscles involved here are your hip abductors (gluteus medius), hip flexors (psoas), hip extensors (gluteus maximus), and hip adductors (especially the adductor magnus). (See Appendix B, page 269, for muscle illustrations.)

The Lower Torso in the Stance Phase

Heel strike: The lower torso, especially the lower abs, should be working hard to pull the body toward the foot, bringing the upper body up over the lower body.

Mid-stance: The lower abs should contract with the mid-back muscles (erector spinae) so that the lowest part of the sandwich system is operative, squeezing together to stabilize the lowest rung of the ladder. The torso begins to twist, motored by the mid-torso (see illustration 3–6).

Pushoff: The lower torso helps to supply the hips with the necessary strength to achieve lift and balance for the next step. The lower torso continues to hold the upper body up over the lower body.

The Mid-torso in the Stance Phase During forward movement, the focal point of body rotation comes from the mid-torso. It's extremely important to understand that the mid-torso is the source of the twist, which should take place at the axis of your body, often referred to as the solar plexus.

Body twist is often lost, especially for people who walk leaning-back. In a flailing attempt to add efficiency to their walks, some people twist artificially by throwing their arms, or sometimes even their shoulders. The correct way to accomplish this important facet of a balanced movement should be to generate the twist from deep inside at around the level of the solar plexus. The arms and shoulders should follow, not cause, the swivel.

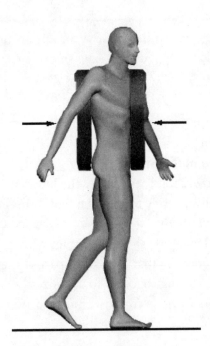

3–6 The sandwich system

Your spine runs down your body from your head to your hips. Think of it as a rod twisting on itself, rotating like a washing machine agitator but without the violent agitation, back and forth with each step. This twisting causes the rest of the body, particularly the parts on the outside, to follow. When the twist comes from deep inside, it appears compact. When it comes from the arms or shoulders, it looks like a robotic flailing motion, which some people misperceive as necessary to generate the necessary body twist.

Heel strike: The mid-torso is preparing for the next step by initiating the first tension required for the twist. The mid-torso also helps keep the upper body up and over the lower body.

Mid-stance: The upper abs and the mid-back muscles (erector spinae) co-contract throughout mid-stance and pushoff, holding on to each other, literally sandwiching everything in between and stabilizing the trunk. At this point, the arms and legs can easily do whatever they want because they have a stable foundation from which to move.

Pushoff: The mid-torso should be helping to lift the body against gravity, which, of course, is doing *its* job of trying to pull you down.

The Upper Torso in the Stance Phase This is the most difficult area when it comes to a balanced Primary Movement Pattern. That's because your head is heavy, and yet it's near the top. In fact, your upper torso has an interesting configuration. It's like your little neck is holding up a bowling ball, with various limbs and other body parts involved in the balancing act. Think of a Christmas tree. If all the ornaments are evenly distributed, happy holidays. But if your Christmas tree stand isn't stable, or if the trunk is already drooping to one side with extra branches and decorations, and then you put a fifteen-pound angel on top, this will bode well for the Grinch.

When the upper torso is forced to compensate for certain oddities down below, it develops its own quirks. I see heads and necks that appear to be growing out in front of the upper torso instead of on top of the body. When I do, I can safely assume that the building blocks down below are experiencing imbalance and that the head is being used as a counterbalance, a bad use for one's head.

Heel strike: The upper rib muscles (both front and back) should pull down, as should the chest muscle (pectoral muscle, or "pecs") on the front and the back shoulder blade muscle (latissimus dorsi, or "lats") on the back. This offsets the lift from the lower and mid-torso. If the twist were not countered in this manner, it would keep on going rather than reset itself for the next twist. Twist emanates from inside, and the shoulder and scapular muscles carry it through and offer balance.

Try taking five steps or so. Notice how, when your right heel strikes, your right shoulder is back and your left shoulder is forward? At that moment your lats on the right are more active, as are your pecs on the left. Notice how, when your right foot is forward, your left arm is as far forward as your right arm is back (at least it should be, both at about 35 degrees from the body's vertical plane). Your lower jaw should be parallel to the ground, even dropped a bit lower, rather than up in the air. A person watching you approach should be able to see the crown of your head. Naturally this test falls flat if that person isn't about your height, but keep in mind that the crown of your head should be facing slightly forward.

Mid-stance: The shoulders, pecs, and lats are coming to a neutral spot where for a split second they join the body in a perpendicular plane. That is, when the body is hanging on one foot, there's a split second when it's all facing front as the two diagonals move simultaneously, actually getting ready to trade places as they pass by each other. At this point the chin, neck, and head are as they were at heel strike. The underside of the nose should be parallel to the floor.

Pushoff: Assuming we're still on the right foot, the right shoulder is pulled back in accordance with the twisting of the rod (spine). Your arms should be energized with activity, too. They're not just along for a free ride. Imagine them pulling the air. They're working as an integral part of this whole-body sport called walking.

• • •

The Swing Phase

The swing phase of a step is comprised of everything your body does from the time your toes leave the floor to the time your heel strikes the ground again. In other words, swing phase is the part of your step when your leg moves through the air.

In addition, you may recall that the function of the swing phase is to shorten your leg so you don't scuff your toes, drag your heels, or have to swing your leg out to clear the ground. The swing phase is also largely responsible for propelling your body forward. Your leg acts a little like a weighted pendulum, except in this case it's abruptly stopped and thrown into reverse halfway through its cycle, which is helped along further by another swinging motion of the upper torso, accomplished with your arms. The intricate interaction of human parts during each step is as mechanically astonishing as sight, yet we take it for granted because at birth the technology was licensed to us for free.

The swing phase is no less amazing, though you might think of a leg moving through the air as nothing too thrilling. The swing phase, however, is extremely important to a balanced movement pattern and is often done inefficiently. The swing phase, unlike the stance phase, is easiest to explain by looking at the feet, ankles, knees, and hips together. Following that comes a description of what the upper half of the body looks like for each part of the step: heel strike, mid-stance, and pushoff.

The Feet, Ankles, Knees, and Hips in the Swing Phase As your heel comes off the ground and the toes bend for pushoff, your entire leg is preparing for flight. When your toes finally leave the ground, they actually lift up before they straighten again, which sends a message to the rest of the leg that starts a chain reaction of bending, shortening, and continued forward momentum.

The toe muscles used to push your leg (and body) off the ground are stretched just prior to pushoff. Stretched muscles always shorten reflexively the other way, like a rubber band springing back to its original shape. The heel, which should remain down as long as possible to optimize stretch, causes other opposing muscles to bend the ankle, which causes the foot to come up. At the same instant, the knee, which was nearly straightened when behind you, goes through the same kind of stretch reflex, which causes the knee to bend. All the major weight-bearing joints (the hips, knees, ankles, and toes) bend after specific opposing muscle groups are stretched. That stretch causes a reflex reaction to shorten again, signaled when the toes complete the pushoff. All these reflexive actions are part of shortening the leg for ground clearance.

> The opposing muscle groups in action here are the psoas versus the gluteus maximus at the hip, hamstrings versus quads at the knee joint, anterior tibialis versus gastrox/soleus at the ankle joint, and flexor digitorum versus extensor digitorum at the toes.

Some of the real pioneers in the special field of movement are Maggie Knott and Dorothy Voss. They incorporated diagonal movement patterns into a masterful combination of exercises that use the stretch reflex to retrain and/or strengthen weak limbs and other body parts. This concept was instrumental in my understanding proper gait and this Primary Movement Balancing system.

The Lower Torso in the Swing Phase The lower torso twists during the swing phase. Earlier in the chapter we asked you to imagine taking hold of a toy doll and twisting her right shoulder back (pushing her left shoulder forward) and her right hip forward (pushing her left hip back). That's the twist I'm talking about. So imagine that the doll has a little springiness to her. When her left foot comes off the ground (it's still behind her), her lower abdominal muscles and her hip flexor muscles would tighten and contract to pull the leg forward.

If those two muscle groups (the lower abs and hip flexors) aren't working well, your hip joints have to work double-time to hold up your entire body. Ouch. The longer you let this go on (walk without proper torso twist), the weaker those two muscle groups get. If you haven't used your lower abs and hip flexors in awhile, it might be harder to introduce the correct torso twist, but you can. Some of my patients erroneously think they were born without the ability to accomplish the torso twist, until they actually do it. The proper lower torso action in the swing phase is for the lower abs and the hip flexors (on the swinging side) to be hard at work.

The Mid-Torso in the Swing Phase I've already mentioned that the mid-torso is your power generator. To help understand how, imagine a line of ice-skaters, arms locked, ready to begin the whip routine. Have you ever been to an ice show and seen a big line of skaters who slowly begin to turn, with the linked arms of the two center skaters as the axis, one facing forward, and one backward, like a huge human propeller? The innermost skaters initiate the entire momentum, followed by the skaters next to them, and expanding outward until the very last skaters get going, and those skaters go the fastest of all. Those last skaters are like your hands, traveling the fastest, all based on the power generated from the middle, and that's your spine. Your erector spinae, or spinal muscles, are the power generators that we tend to overlook because they don't show on the outside of the body. The spinal muscles tighten around the spine hard to create the very first impulse and the power to start the twist. The mid-torso also has the extremely important job of lifting the upper body so that it isn't compressing the lower body as gravity would have it. The balance and efficiency of the upper abs and the upper back muscles are the sources of power in your walk, though many people unknowingly sit back and let the hips and legs do all the work, causing structural weakness.

The Upper Torso in the Swing Phase The most important thing the upper torso does is to keep the shoulders down in spite of the fact that the mid-torso, lower torso, and hips are all lifting like crazy against gravity. Many people try to use their shoulders to hold up their bodies, thus offering the odd, stiff appearance of being carried around on a coat hanger. Patients with shoulders that appear to come up to their ears typically say they carry tension in their shoulders and necks—no surprise to me! Well-balanced bodies might have tension in their necks and shoulders, too, but when they walk with structural balance, their muscular tension dissolves.

It's also important to know what role the arms play in the swing phase. Many people walk carrying their arms as if they're some weird appendages that are just along for the ride. Wrong. Walking is a whole-body sport, and the arms play an important role in forward propulsion. Although the trunk is twisting, the arms shouldn't swing around the body. They should move in a straight line, parallel to the direction of travel. When the arms are used correctly, they help stop the body's twist with some degree of muscle tension at the end of the swing. Without the arms as a counterbalance, the powerful inner momentum that generates the twist might have us spin around too far with each step. Have you ever seen someone whose hands seem to fly up too high?

In addition, the head and neck should be pulling up, but just to the extent that a person looking directly at your height would see the crown of your head, as was stated earlier. A soft lift of the head works best, without tension or rigidity.

The Whole Picture

I've broken down the act of walking into two phases (swing and stance) and divided each phase into physical segments (feet, ankles, knees, hips, and lower/middle/upper torso), and we've further described what's expected from each for a proper gait. Putting the pieces together to formulate your own balanced movement pattern is coming up next, right after the analysis of your current gait. I don't expect you to have mastered *any* techniques yet, but it's important to get a *feel* for where we're headed with a proper gait.

The references to muscles and joints in this chapter should help you be aware of what's going on in your body as you walk. Use your muscles, notice the tension, and feel that moment of balance that comes with each step. Most important, experience the work going on as your stomach muscles and back muscles sandwich your torso together with strength.

After you've developed habits that are conducive to a proper gait, you can stop thinking about walking. Your new walk will happen subconsciously, replacing your old walk. Until that time, however, every step you take is an opportunity to strengthen yourself, to feel how you move around, and to sense what constitutes a balanced Primary Movement Pattern. You are about to walk yourself well!

CUSTOMIZE YOUR ANTIPAIN STRATEGY

EVALUATE YOURSELF AND DETERMINE WHICH GAIT CORRECTIONS YOU NEED

T his is the part of the book you've been waiting for—the part about you. This chapter helps you determine the specific gait corrections and exercises you need to walk away from pain.

The first step is to determine what your Primary Movement Pattern looks like at this point in time. It is extremely important to note, however, that the process of self evaluation, not to mention the implementation of your gait corrections, has a prerequisite: you must understand the first three chapters of this book.

Removing (and preventing) structural pain requires that you know what structural stability is all about. If you don't have a conceptual grasp of where you're headed, the upcoming path to structural stability will be hazy, and you may do the gait corrections and exercises incorrectly. On the other hand, when you have a clear picture of how and why your body performs so much more efficiently (and painlessly) when it's in structural balance, the road map sharpens into focus.

As you proceed, keep in mind what you've read so far and constantly ask yourself if you're adhering to the basics of human motion as presented in the preceding chapters of this book. When you do that, the ensuing gait corrections and exercises will be far more enlightening and productive.

ARE YOU READY TO PROCEED?

We've devised a little test for you. Ask yourself these true-or-false questions to see if you are ready to proceed:

1. It's highly unlikely that a childhood ankle injury could cause shoulder pain later in life.
   ○ T   ○ F

2. By using the well-designed structure of your hip joints to hold you up and balance you as you walk, you can avoid structural vulnerability and pain.
   ○ T   ○ F

3. It was Boone, and not a preexisting condition, that caused Terry's accident and subsequent back pain.
   ○ T   ○ F

4. The best way to attain good posture is to keep your chest up and your shoulders back.
   ○ T   ○ F

5. You conserve energy and attain greater structural efficiency if you lock your knees when you stand or walk.
   ○ T   ○ F

6. Your arms do not play a role during the act of walking.
   ○ T   ○ F

7. The term "stance phase" refers to when you stand with both feet on the ground, arms down, facing forward.

　○ T　　　　　　　　○ F

If you answered "true" to any of the questions above, you have become overly zealous about your prospects of walking away from pain. The correct answer to all the questions is "false." Your anxiousness is admirable, but you will discover that you need to understand the theory and methodology before you practice the concepts described in this book. Please go back and reread the first part, or at least read enough to figure out why you answered the question(s) incorrectly.

If you answered "false" to all the questions above, good job! You're ready for the self-evaluation profile.

WHAT TO DO BEFORE YOUR SELF-EVALUATION PROFILE

To complete your self-evaluation, you need to prepare. First, we're going to assume that you have access to a full-length mirror. Second, although you *can* satisfactorily complete this evaluation without the help of another person, there are certain aspects of how you walk that make another set of eyes helpful.

You should plan to wear light, form-fitting clothing, or if your spirit allows, wear even less, because you will need to see your body. Don't wear loose-fitting clothes. As you proceed with the self-evaluation, you'll observe certain body parts that you frequently hide during the winter months.

EVALUATION GROUND RULES

These questions will require that you stand, or walk, or sometimes just think about something. When you stand, stand with your feet apart as you normally would, as if you were in line at the movies. In other words, stand the way you do when you're not thinking about standing; nobody is watching you, and you're just hanging around standing.

When you walk, walk at a normal pace, as if you were walking to your local theater to see a movie, for which you are not late. Again, walk the way you do when you're not thinking about walking and nobody is watching.

Almost all of the evaluation consists of yes-or-no questions. Sometimes a question will pertain to body parts of which you have two, a right and a left, and therefore there will be a box for each. Your right leg might do something different from your left. Don't assume they're the same. When you get to those types of questions, we'll prompt you for two answers like this:

◯ Left   ◯ Right

If there's no "left" or "right," that means you don't have to worry about distinguishing between sides.

If you're asked about something that has an inner or outer part—your foot, for example—just fill in the appropriate word ("inner" or "outer") so you can remember your observation.

Each question is preceded by a symbol that indicates if you should be walking, standing, looking in a mirror, being observed, or just ruminating, as follows:

    •••• = walking (walk around and look at or feel what's going on to determine an accurate answer)

    ↑↑ = standing (stand up and look at or feel what's going on to arrive at your answer)

    👁 = mirror (use a mirror to observe yourself)

⊖ = being observed (for answering this question you can benefit from, or need the assistance of, someone else)

♀ = ruminating (make a mental observation by visualizing, listening to, or recalling something about yourself)

Most of the information you'll need will be collected by looking at
yourself or feeling how your body works. Sometimes you will actually
look at yourself (maybe with a mirror), or you will just mentally
observe (visualize, listen to, or recall) some aspect of your gait or your
body. It's easy.

As for soliciting the help of another person, remember that you
can do this all by yourself. But you will benefit from a second opinion
on some things, and a few things are just too weird to try on your
own (fortunately, there are only a couple of those). Trying to figure
out how you appear from behind as you walk, for example, is horribly
challenging without someone's help (or a video camera).

Not Answering All the Questions Is Okay

If you have trouble answering a question, don't be overly concerned.
Some questions may be difficult because this analytical experience is
new for you. If you're asked "Do you carry your weight in a certain
part of your body?" for example, you may raise an eyebrow and
scratch your perplexed head. Try to answer as best you can. If you
draw a blank or can't answer at all, don't worry; go on to the next
question. Even with an incomplete evaluation, you'll still have
enough information to establish a pattern and a corrective solution.

All the questions have something to do with how you hold yourself
upright against the earth's gravitational pull. Staying upright starts
with your feet, your structural foundation, which is where most structural deviations begin. So with your connection to earth in mind
(your talented feet), that's where you'll start your self-evaluation.

TRANSLATING YOUR EVALUATION TO SPECIFIC GAIT CORRECTIONS

If you answer yes to a question, or if it applies to your particular condition or anatomy, you need the correction indicated at the end of that section (each gait correction is numbered so you can find them easily in Chapter 5). If you answer no to a question, or if the question doesn't apply to you, skip that question and go on to the next.

YOUR SELF-EVALUATION

1. Is your heel strike off center?

⬤⬤ As your heel touches the ground, does it first touch on the inner or outer edge? Walk around a bit and feel which part of your heel contacts the ground first. Walk away from a friend and have him or her watch you from behind (to see where your heel strikes). Does your friend see your heel strike on the inside or outside of your foot?

Left: ○ Inside   ○ Outside   Right: ○ Inside   ○ Outside

꙳ Another way to tell if your heel strike is off center is to check your shoes. Are the heels of your shoes more worn out on the inside or the outside?

Left: ○ Inside   ○ Outside   Right: ○ Inside   ○ Outside

Effect: Remember that your feet carry your body's entire weight, and they'll do it best when your base of support provides balance and stability. The balancing act of walking starts with a centered heel strike. If yours is off center, that precarious foundation will have a ripple effect straight up through your entire body. I frequently tell patients that when their heel strike is off center, they're out of balance before their foot even hits the ground.

See Gait Correction 1.1.

2. Do your ankles roll inward?

↑↑ Do your feet roll in at the ankles (pronate) so that your inner ankle bones look like they lean slightly down toward the floor?

　○ Left　　　　　○ Right

•••☜ 👀 As you're walking, do you feel your weight shift inward toward the inside of your ankle(s) at mid-step? As you walk toward a mirror, do you see your ankles roll in a bit with each step? Are they

4–1 (a) Ankles straight (b) Ankles rolled in

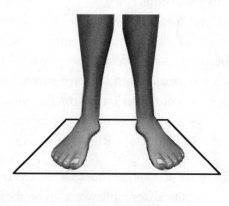

(a)

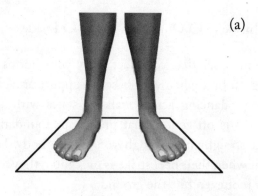

(b)

rolled in throughout the entire step? (Having someone watch you can help with this one.)

    ⃝ Left   ⃝Right

Effect: When your weight shifts to the inside of your ankles, it sets off a chain reaction that starts at the feet and moves up through your knees, hips, back, shoulders, and neck, and you'll automatically lean back. Centering your ankle distributes your weight evenly and helps balance your body. When moving in balance, your body uses all the necessary muscles (in the correct proportions) to naturally reduce structural vulnerabilities.

See Gait Correction 2.1.

3. How do your feet participate in propelling you forward?

👁.👄 When you walk, do you pick your feet up in a flat-footed manner, sort of like a penguin? Do your calves feel relaxed and flaccid as you pick up your feet? Are your inner calves skinnier or flabbier than your outer calves (facing a mirror, do your inner and outer calves appear to be equally proportionate)? If you answered yes to any question above, you're probably underworking the muscles that should be propelling you forward.

Do you take relatively short steps, as opposed to having a long stride? A short stride can mean you're not bending your toes (and working your muscles) to create a longer step as you push off with your foot. Check the toe boxes of your older shoes. If they aren't wrinkled at the toes, that's a sign that you don't bend your toes when you walk.

Women: when you walk in high heels, does your foot, ankle, or heel wobble a bit with each step? If so, this also indicates that your feet are failing to participate properly in propelling you forward.

Effect: Bending your toes at pushoff is important for propelling you forward. You should feel your weight move all the way into your big and middle toes as you push off. Your toes bend, your calves tighten, and your bun muscles should all go into action. This is accomplished most efficiently by keeping your heel down for a split second longer, by taking a little longer stride, and by bending your toes at the end of each stance phase.

See Gait Corrections 1.3 and 4.3.

.••° During the swing phase do your toes move very little (or not at all)? They should lift so you can feel them touch the top inside of the toe box of your shoes as you walk. Try lifting your toenails so they touch the top inside of your shoe. That's where your toes should be as your foot travels through the air.

☞•••°6ə Another test is to have your partner sit in a chair while you walk toward him or her. Ask your partner if he or she can see the bottoms of your shoes as you approach. As you walk toward a mirror, can you see the bottoms of your feet? Or, find a hard surface to walk on so you can listen to your footsteps. Do your feet make a *ker-plunk* sound as your heel steps first and the ball of your foot plops down second? If so, you are not holding your toes up correctly. When your toes are active, there should be little or no sound.

Effect: Your toes do much more than provide balance during the stance phase. They play a big role in your swing phase, too, as they contribute to your forward motion. You have to lift your toes and feet in order to have that important "split second of balance" that will help strengthen your entire body as you walk (we'll explain this concept later in the book).

See Gait Correction 2.2.

4. Are your footsteps narrower than your hip joints?
For this question, you need a straight line about fifteen feet long. You can use a preexisting line on a level surface, like the line on a tile floor. Or you can put down a piece of tape to make a temporary line (make sure you don't mess up a nice floor with sticky adhesive). An outside observer comes in handy for this one, or you can set up a mirror at the end of the line.

👁●⦁•⦁69 Walk normally down the line and determine how far to either side of the line your foot lands. Keep the line in front of you, centered with your nose as you walk. Don't walk on the line like it's a sobriety test; walk normally with your head up (don't look down to calculate the distance, because looking down makes you lean back—use a mirror or take short little glances down). Estimate how many inches away from the center line the innermost edge of your heel lands.

Other options: You can use the preexisting lines on a level sidewalk. Step in some water and then walk down the line, head up, as described above. Nice footprints, eh? Measure from the innermost edge of your footprint to the center line.

The most rudimentary method is to simply imagine a line running from your nose, through your navel, and onto the floor. That's your center line. Then estimate your foot width from the center line, or look at your feet as you walk toward a mirror to estimate the distance from your midline to your feet.

If the inner edge of one or both feet comes to within two inches of the line (or touches, or even crosses over, the line), then the width of your step needs to be increased to improve the stability of your footing.

Effect: If your base of support is too narrow, your balance will be impaired and you'll have to waddle to stay on your feet. Even if the waddle is indiscernible, your stability will be like a bowling pins—wobbly. If one or both feet cross the midline, or even if they come close to the midline, you are a candidate for back or leg pain. Here's your solution:

If both your feet land less than two inches from your center line when you walk, you need Correction 4.1. If they cross over your center line, you may have noticed that your feet scuff together as you walk. You definitely need Gait Correction 4.1.

If only your left foot comes within two inches of the line, or crosses over it, see Gait Correction 4.2L.

If only your right foot comes within two inches of the line, or crosses over it, see Gait Correction 4.2R.

5. Do your feet turn out too much?

👁.•⁀• Are one or both feet turned out more than 15 or 20 degrees? Take a look at illustration 4-2 to see about how much turnout you should have. How do your feet compare? Walk toward a mirror to see how much foot turnout you have.

Effect: If your feet turn out too much, your hips, knees, and feet naturally tend to develop musculoskeletal weakness that can lead to pain in the hips, knees, feet, neck, and back.

If your turnout is greater than 20 degrees, see Gait Correction 1.2.

6. Do you lock your knees when you stand or walk?

👁↑↑.•⁀• Looking at a side view of yourself standing normally, are your legs perfectly straight? Are your knees locked or even hyperextended (bowed back)? When you walk, does it feel like you're walking on peg legs, with your knees locked straight at the point of heel strike or at midstance? Do your knees get achy when you walk or stand a lot?

Effect: When you walk with locked knees, the muscles around your knees get weaker, plus you tend to lean back. Your knees should be slightly bent and feel springy when you walk. They should be spongy or soft, even when you stand.

See Gait Correction 3.1.

7. Do you balance with each step?

👣.•⁀• While your weight is all on one foot, imagine freezing in mid-step for just a split second. Would you feel unstable and/or like you might fall over? You should feel stable, like you could freeze and stay well balanced on one foot with your weight mostly forward.

Effect: A balanced walk is crucial for developing the muscles that keep you out of structural trouble. Using your muscles to balance

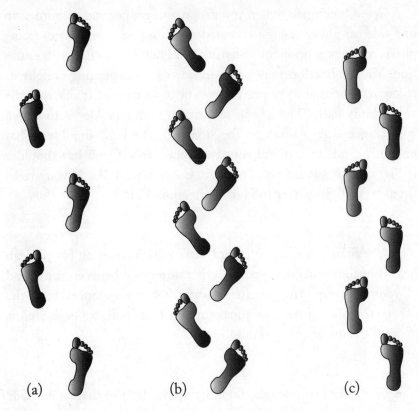

(a)   (b)   (c)

4–2 (a) Correct: feet turned out at fifteen to twenty degrees (b) Incorrect: feet turned out too far (c) Incorrect: no turn out at all

yourself with each step is best accomplished by extending your swing phase (slow it down and make it last longer).

See Gait Corrections 2.2 and 4.4.

8. Do your two sides work together evenly?

☞↑↑Is one of your shoulders higher than the other? If so, do you carry anything on a regular basis, like a briefcase, shoulder bag, or toolbox? Be aware of your daily habits. Do you always give one side a certain task or unique position, something the other side doesn't get to do?

Effect: Once again, when you assign a disproportionate burden to one side, or always assign repeated tasks to one side, that overemphasis may cause problems. Sharing sides helps neutralize this situation. Your correction may be as simple as redistributing weight or changing work habits to prevent overtaxing a particular side or individual body parts. The key to lowering a high shoulder is to widen your stance (step wider) on the side with the high shoulder. That naturally tends to equalize your two shoulders. If your left shoulder is higher, you should refer to Gait Correction 4.2L. If your right shoulder is higher, refer to Gait Correction 4.2R.

•••When you walk on a hard surface with shoes on (so you can hear your footsteps), can you discern a difference between the sound of your two steps that might indicate that one is longer than the other? You should hear an equal rhythm that indicates each step is about the same length and duration.

Effect: Your two sides should function similarly so that no one side gets an unfair burden. Structural pain can be the result of years of lopsided movements, even when one side is only slightly overstressed.
See Gait Correction 4.3.

☞↑↑When you go to the tailor or try on pants, does one of your pant legs seem shorter than the other? Is one of your hips a little (or a lot) higher than the other? (That could be why your pant legs aren't even.) Your situation should be remedied by lowering the higher hip.

Effect: The key to lowering a high hip is to widen your stance on the opposite side of the hip that's too high. Widening the opposite foot tends to bring down the higher hip.

If your left hip is higher (your left pant leg is shorter), see Gait Correction 4.2R.

If your right hip is higher (your right pant leg is shorter), see Gait Correction 4.2L.

👁•• ••Do you punch one hip out to the side farther than the other as you walk? Use a mirror, or have someone help you with this one.

Effect: Generally, only one hip tends to have that Mae West jut. For a balanced gait, you need to equalize both hips by reducing that hip slide. (If both hips slide out to the side when you walk, you're leaning back and you need Gait Correction 6.1.)

If your left hip juts out, see Gait Correction 4.2R.

If your right hip juts out, see Gait Correction 4.2L.

9. Do you sit back into your hip joints?

💡👁↑↑When you stand casually is your weight more toward your heels than toward the balls of your feet? From a side view, does your head appear forward on your body? Does standing make your back tired, or does walking for an extended period of time make your back achy? These are the most common signs of someone who "sits in their hips." Another typical indicator is that from a side view your belly may appear to protrude, even though you may be thin. People who are not overweight tend to pop out their bellies simply because their natural posture is to lean back. How does your stomach look from the side?

Effect: If you answered yes to any of these questions, you undoubtedly sit in your hips, and you need to change that by shifting your weight slightly forward onto the balls of your feet, where it belongs.

See Gait Correction 6.1.

☞↑↑ Does your belly pop out every time you inhale? Do you feel or see your chest and ribs move up toward your chin each time you inhale? The way you breathe will either help or impair your ability to attain a structurally sound gait.

Effect: The key to proper breathing, at least as it interplays with the way you walk, is to learn to breathe sideways. Breathing sideways (which is explained further in Gait Correction 6.2) allows you to stay forward. Breathing into your belly, or up into your chest, throws your weight back.

See Gait Correction 6.2.

Some people have been taught to tuck their buns neatly under so they don't show too much, and that leads to sitting in your hips and leaning back.

☞•• Do your pants seem too big or baggy where your buns should be? When you walk, do you feel your weight stay in the center of your body with each step, as opposed to correctly shifting from hip to hip? If you *do* shift from hip to hip, do you slide so far out that you have that Mae West hip jut?

☞↑↑ Does your lower back seem to be too straight, as if you're missing your own buttocks? Take a look at illustration 4-3 and compare it to your profile. Have you lost that natural curve?

Effect: You depend on your hip joints too much for support instead of using your muscles to stabilize your lower torso. As you walk, you need to shift your weight from hip to hip with your weight forward and untuck your buns in order to regain the natural curve of your lower spine.

See Gait Corrections 5.1 and 5.2.

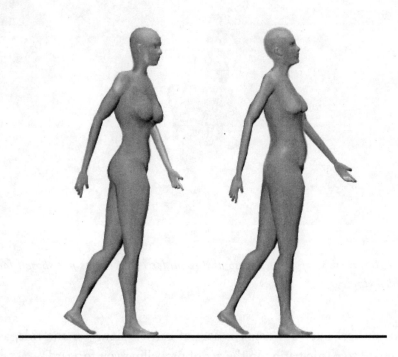

4–3 (a) Correct: normal curve of the back when body is forward (b) Incorrect: curve is lost when leaning back

👁•◦•👣 If your kneecaps were headlights, would your beams point slightly in at each other or straight ahead (as opposed to aiming slightly out-ward like they should)? Does one kneecap point in or straight ahead?

See Gait Correction 3.2.

10. 👁•◦•👣👣 Does your torso remain inactive as you walk and just tag along for the ride?

•◦•👣 Do your shoulders face straight ahead in the direction you are walking, as opposed to turning to face each step? Do your shoulders move slightly up and down instead of twisting horizontally?

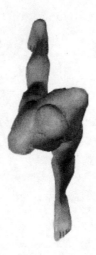

4–4 Aerial view of correct torso and shoulder twist (arms not shown for added clarity)

Do you feel like your trunk is sort of carried along for the ride, as opposed to participating in the act of propelling you forward?

Take a look at illustration 4.4 and determine whether you have proper trunk rotation. If your trunk doesn't twist properly as you walk, you are pulling your weight instead of using it to propel you forward.

Effect: Your upper body is not cargo. It needs to actively participate along with your legs and everything else as you walk. It's important that you rotate your shoulders so that they face each step forward. Remember, walking is a whole-body sport.

See Gait Correction 6.3.

👁👆👆•‿•👂💡 Do your shoulders roll forward a little or are they slouched forward most of the time? Do your shoulders move up and down with each step you take? Do you carry tension around in your shoulders? Do you ever feel like your shoulders are up to your ears, and if so, do you revert back to a slouched, seemingly more relaxed, posture after a while? Were you taught that good posture was synony-mous with "chest up, shoulders back"?

Effect: It appears that your shoulders have a little attitude, and it may be getting in the way of a balanced, sturdy gait. If you answered yes to any of these questions, it indicates that the position of your shoulders and chest are "up and out" instead of "back and down," where they should be. Pull your chest, shoulders, and back down, and keep your shoulders level (your shoulder rotation should be horizon-tal, not vertical).

See Gait Correction 6.4.

11. Do your arms get a free ride, too?

👁••‘• Are your arms somewhat passive as you walk? Do you carry them around like big summer sausages? If you do use your arms, do they swing around or away from your body as you walk? Do you walk with the palms of your hands facing back?

Effect: Your arms are yet another integral part of your gait. Use them, don't carry them. Adjust the angle of your arm swing and let your thumbs lead the way to the front as your pinkies lead the way to the rear.

See Gait Corrections 7.1, 7.2, 7.3, and 7.4.

12. Do you walk with your head slightly forward?

👁••‘• Do you walk with your head up, a little forward, and with your chin slightly out in front? When you walk toward a mirror, can you see the crown of your head?

Effect: Yes, your head is actually just along for the ride, but like any good passenger, where and how it sits makes a big difference.

Your head should be up but back, with your chin and your eyes point-ing slightly down. If you cannot see the crown of your head as you approach a mirror, your head is most likely too far forward and tilted up instead of down.

See Gait Correction 8.

⧉ 5 ⧉

GAIT CORRECTIONS

SIMPLE WAYS TO CORRECT YOUR WALK

Congratulations! You're ready to take your first steps toward structural stability and away from pain. The most direct route calls for your full participation. That means practicing your gait corrections every day. Fortunately, that doesn't mean extensive, rigorous, or time-consuming workouts. They're short, but they do require dedicated concentration so that you can experience meaningful change.

WHICH CORRECTIONS TO DO, HOW OFTEN, AND FOR HOW LONG

Your personal profile (as determined by your self-evaluation in the previous chapter) indicates the gait corrections you need most. It's extremely important to *read through all of the corrections* at least once, however, to make sure you are not missing an opportunity to correct some aspect of your gait that somehow got overlooked in your personal profile. Since all the gait corrections work together as part of a single system, it's wise to know about all of them. Then focus your attention on the exercises indicated in your personal profile, starting with the lowest numbers first.

Most people like to work on three gait corrections at a time. Some prefer five or six; others, one or two. After you read this chapter and all the corrections, begin by rereading and implementing the gait corrections indicated on your personal profile list. If your list includes gait corrections 1.1, 1.3, 2.1, 3.2, 4.2L, 4.4, 5.2, 6.3, 6.4, and 8, for example, you would begin with the three lowest numbers (in this case, corrections 1.1, 1.3, and 2.1) and concentrate on those three corrections until you feel confident that you have grasped the concepts and incorporated those corrections into your new gait. That can take a few days or a few weeks—it's up to you.

Note: If gait correction 6.1 is on your list, include it as one of the first gait corrections you work on and master it before you replace it with another gait correction. You may find you want to go back to it periodically, too.

Notice that the lower-numbered gait corrections correspond to the lower parts of your body. Number 1 deals with your feet, and gait correction number 8 deals with your head. It's important to incorporate these corrections from the bottom up. Ground level is where the balancing act begins. You need a sturdy foundation. As you progress upward from your feet with more and more gait corrections, this entire system will make more and more sense.

The time spent on gait corrections (and exercises and stretching) varies among people. The recommended time for walking practice is five minutes, four times a day. You can speed up the process if you practice more. You may feel real good about one correction before you're finished with the other two, in which case you might add a new correction in the place of the one you've mastered. If done too fast, or too much, some of them may cause a little soreness. That's okay, and the discomfort will subside as you get stronger. Slow down a bit if necessary.

CORRESPONDING GAIT CORRECTIONS
AND EXERCISES

You'll see that most gait corrections have supportive corrections listed along with them. These are secondary corrections that will make the ones you're working on easier and more sustainable. It's totally up to you whether or not you decide to use the supportive gait corrections.

You may find exercises listed along with the gait corrections, too. You will lock in the corrections more rapidly and benefit more permanently by doing the corresponding exercises for each correction. Both the strengthening and stretching exercises associated with each gait correction are extremely beneficial and highly recommended. You can spend as little as ten minutes a day and as much as an hour a day on these exercises. Your choice will determine the speed at which you assimilate the gait corrections.

WHEN AM I FINISHED WITH THE PROGRAM
FOR GOOD?

Working through the gait corrections can take weeks or months, depending on your particular situation and your practice routine. Eventually the gait corrections will be so firmly built into your movement pattern that you won't have to think about them anymore! You will use your corrected gait automatically because it feels better. Your new walk will permanently replace your old walk, and every step you take will be a strengthening one that balances your body. At some point you'll try to remember what your old walking style looked like. You'll probably try to imitate that old style. This can be an exhilarating source of free entertainment, because you'll have the hardest time remembering how you walked before, and it simply won't be as comfortable.

In some ways, you'll always be working on these corrections. I am.

Strains, stresses, and pains pop up, and they may get factored into your Primary Movement Pattern. You will want to use these techniques to gently rebalance your gait.

CHARTING YOUR PROGRAM
AND PROGRESS

To simplify organizing your gait corrections and exercise routine, it's a good idea to chart out where you're headed. In Appendix A (page 263) you'll find a fill-in-the-blank chart that you can use to track your course. (You can also make your own even bigger; just follow this as an example.) There's also a sample chart that shows how one person mapped out the first few weeks of gait corrections and exercises.

List the first correction you've chosen to work on under the column headed "Week 1." Underneath that, list any other gait corrections you plan on tackling in your first week.

In the strengthening exercise chart, list the strengthening exercises that correspond to the gait correction you're working on. That goes under "Week 1," too. (There's no need to chart out the stretching exercises, but you can if you want to.) When the second week rolls around, if you have not mastered a gait correction listed under "Week 1," list it again under "Week 2." When you feel you've mastered that gait correction, write in a new correction.

As for updating your exercise routine, as you update your chart to include more and more exercises, you may want to continue doing the ones you liked. As for the ones you found hardest to do, you may want to continue them also, since that's a sign that they were beneficial. If you had trouble with a particular gait correction you may want to choose a different exercise. Since nobody has a body exactly like yours, be aware of what's working and don't be afraid to alter your course. After a while you won't really need the chart, or you may just glance back at it to refresh your memory.

VERBALIZE YOUR GAIT CORRECTIONS AS YOU DO THEM

As you practice, the system works best if you verbally describe the gait corrections to yourself as you do them. It's like a mantra. You might say to yourself as you walk, "Up and over" (and check yourself to make sure you *are* up and over), "Unlock the knees" (check your knees), and "Widen the base" (check your feet to make sure they're under your hip joints). Verbalize your corrections and confirm them while you're doing them over and over throughout your practice.

In the beginning, most people repeat their verbal reinforcements for only short periods of time, and then they start thinking about dinner, or picking up their dry cleaning, and *poof*—there go the verbal reinforcements. Expect lapses. As with any other contemplative or meditative focus, gently steer yourself back to the process at hand without belittling or badgering yourself for wandering off. You've lost nothing but a few seconds. Many patients tell me that their practice sessions are an oasis for recharging their batteries during or after a hectic day of hustle and bustle. Your sessions can actually be quite rejuvenating.

GET READY, GET SET . . .

Wait. Don't go yet. Every time you are about to begin a gait correction session, you need to prepare physically and mentally. The mental part involves visualizing what you're about to do before you do it. The physical part means getting into the appropriate starting position by following the instructions listed below. (These preparations are simplified gait corrections, which you'll understand after you read this entire chapter, and they're applicable to some degree for everyone.) So, each gait correction session should start with the following:

- Lift your body up and over.
- Unlock your knees.
- Bring your weight to the front of your feet.
- Bring your chest down and lower your chin.
- Visualize widened steps and horizontal shoulder rotation.
- Take a big sideways breath.
- Go!

Important: Remember that this system works best when you do it in short sessions, four times a day, *evenly spread out.* If you're rushed, spend just three minutes per session, but squeeze in all four sessions. Don't do one long session that lasts twenty minutes and then not think about it again for the rest of the day. You're attempting to retrain a very powerfully ingrained system, and that takes continuous repetition, best accomplished by interjecting lots of mini-sessions throughout your day. Pretty soon you'll feel your body gravitate to your new walk without thinking—it will just feel superior.

Here is a list of all the Gait Corrections, followed by the page number on which each one is explained.

GAIT CORRECTIONS

1. Feet

1.1. Center your heel strike. Foot pronation signals your body to begin a chain reaction that forces you to lean back. So if your heel first touches the ground off center, you probably lean back when you walk. As we've mentioned many times throughout this book, leaning back is the biggest cause of structural vulnerabilities. An off-center heel strike starts the foot pronation, so centering your heel strike helps prevent leaning back.

If your heel strike is off to one side, one of the easiest ways to center it is to aim to have your heel strike on the other side. So if you normally touch the ground first with the outside of your heel, for example, aim to touch the ground with the inside of your heel. The resulting heel strike will probably end up somewhere in the middle. That's what you're aiming for, the middle.

Note: Oddly enough, the same thing often results whether your heel strikes to the outside or to the inside: foot pronation. Both deviations need the same correction, a centered heel strike, although how you accomplish that is a little different for each. Use this correction and either supportive correction 4.1 or 1.2.

OUTSIDE HEEL STRIKERS: One of the best ways to learn how to center your heel strike is to increase the width of your step by widening the distance between your feet as you walk. Widening your stance naturally causes your heel to strike more toward the middle. Refer to Gait Correction 4.1 or 1.2 and work on it simultaneously with this correction.

Strengthening exercises: Dial Outs, Hip Flexors, Low Ab Knee Switchers, Toes Feet/Feet Toes, Fish Feet (Strengthening Exercises are located in Chapter 6.)
Stretching exercises: Sitting Stretch Routine (Stretching Exercises are located in Chapter 7.)

INSIDE HEEL STRIKERS: One of the best ways to center your heel strike is to pull your heels out. Refer to Gait Correction 1.2 (the next one) and work on it simultaneously with this correction (1.1).

Strengthening exercises: Knee/Toe, Low Ab Knee Switchers, Toes Feet/Feet Toes, Fish Feet
Stretching exercises: Supine Stretch Routine, Wall Stretch Routine

1.2. Pull your heels out for the proper herringbone effect. Adjust your step by pulling your heels out to emulate the footprints in illustration 5-1(a) (mild herringbone pattern). This is the optimal position for healthy feet. But sometimes feet get too herringboned. More than a slight herringbone effect (anything greater than 15 or 20 degrees of toe turnout) is too much and indicates that you should move your heels farther out (rather than moving your toes in, which might tend to adversely narrow the width of your step).

Supportive Gait corrections: 1.3, 2.1 (1.3 will force you to use your hamstrings more.)
Strengthening exercises: Dial Outs, Sitting Hip Flexors, Low Ab Knee Switchers, Standing Hamstrings

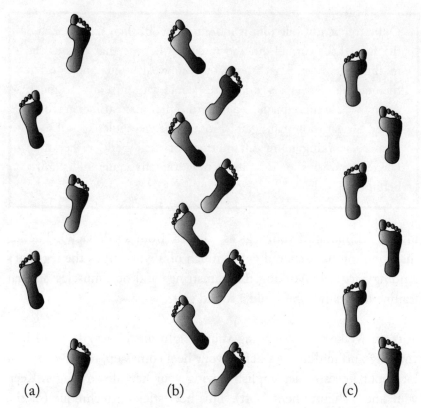

5–1 (a) Correct herringbone pattern (b) Too much turnout (c) Not enough turnout

Stretching exercises: Sitting Stretch Routine (modify this exercise so that you turn your bent knee in instead of out)

1.3. Leave your heels down longer. Imagine having bubblegum stuck to the heels of your shoes so that each time you take a step your heel sticks to the ground a little. That's the feeling you want as you leave your heels down a split second longer with each step you take. When your heels stay down a little longer it forces you to balance and use your hamstrings a little more, and that makes you stronger. It also causes you to walk with your legs under and slightly behind you, where they belong.

Another practical approach to leaving your heel down longer

> Quite frequently, one foot is more turned out than the other, and the foot that's turned out too much is the one that crosses the midline the most. That's typically your weaker side and is often the one that develops sciatic pain. People who turn out too much often overuse their quads and underuse their hamstrings in what's called a "quad-dominant gait." From a side view, it looks as if their legs are working more out in front of their body, rather than where the work should be happening, directly under and slightly behind the body.

involves thinking of your legs as scissors (from a side view). The leg that's pulling back should get as much of a workout as the leg that's striding forward. Working the hamstrings and bun muscles on that trailing leg really helps build a sound gait.

Note: Make sure you bring your weight all the way forward into your big and middle toes before your heel comes up, too, and do not lock your knees to accomplish leaving your heel down longer. Keep your knees slightly bent (soft). This heel-sticking technique (or the scissors technique) needs to work in conjunction with shoulder rotation and torso twisting—very important!

Supportive Gait corrections: 4.3 and 6.3
Strengthening exercises: Alphabet, Toes Feet/Feet Toes, Standing Hip Flexors, Low Ab Knee Switchers, Standing Balance, Tiptoes, Slo-Mo Walking, Hip Extensions
Stretching exercises: Calf Stretch on Wall, Hip Flexor Stretch

2. Ankles

2.1. During midstance, shift your weight to the outsides of your feet. If your weight tends to shift to the inside of your ankle(s) during midstance, you pronate—and you need to compensate for it by shifting your weight a little toward the outside of your foot during midstance. You don't want *all* your weight *on* the outside of your foot, but you should feel your weight move along the inner rim of the outside of your foot. This will help distribute your weight evenly in the middle of your ankle.

Note: Some patients have a tough time with this correction. It's difficult, so don't worry about not getting it perfect at first. Any bit of improvement in your ankle position, however slight, will have a big impact on the rest of your body. The key to strengthening is to systematically challenge your muscles to a new level, and that process may not be comfortable. The supportive corrections listed below (aimed at the knees) will make this ankle correction much easier to accomplish.

Supportive Gait corrections: 3.1, 3.2
Strengthening exercises: Knee/Toe, Standing Sartorius, Towel Scrunches
Stretching exercises: Sitting Stretch Routine, Wall Stretch Routine

2.2. Hold your toes up longer during the swing phase. Remember that the swing phase is everything that happens between the time your toes go airborne until the heel of your same foot strikes the

5–2 Correct weight-bearing surfaces

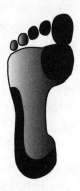

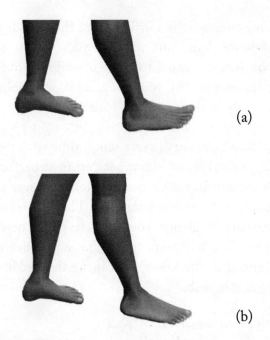

(a)

(b)

5–3 (a) Correct: toe tendons exposed, showing active foot (b) Incorrect: no tendons exposed, showing inactive foot

ground again. You need to flex your toes toward the sky as your foot swings through the air.

Note how, during the swing phase, your foot can travel through the air like a clump (toes passive) or with tension (toes active). The way you can tell if your toes are up and active is that when walking barefoot you will be able to see the tendons of your toes. You'll also notice that you have a much lighter heel strike.

Take off your shoe and sock, and try "holding up" just your big and middle toes. The others may go up, too. See the tendons pop up as you pull your toes back? That's the toe activity you want as you stride forward during the swing phase.

To make sure you're accomplishing this correctly, try to feel your toes touch the top of the inside of your shoe when you walk. Pretend that you are walking toward a mirror, and with each step try to see the bottoms of your shoes (or the soles of your feet) in the mirror for just a fraction of a second. Even if you have on shoes (hard shoes, noncarpeted floor), your foot strike will be silent if your toes are operating correctly.

Note: Each one of your little footsteps carries the entire weight of your body like a controlled balancing act. Recognize that your feet are as dexterous as your hands, except they're designed for balancing instead of for gripping things. Use your muscles to control the balance. When you do, every step becomes an exercise that builds the muscles you need to reduce structural vulnerabilities and pain.

Supportive Gait corrections: 2.1
Strengthening exercises: Alphabet, Toes Feet/Feet Toes, Heel Walk
Stretching exercises: Wall Stretch Routine, Supine Stretch Routine

3. Knees

3.1. Unlock your knees. Your knees are not meant to be straightened out all the way (locked) as you walk or stand. They should be very slightly bent and springy. People who lean back when they walk often do so because their knees are locked.

When you soften your knees, your legs automatically start the process of shifting your weight to the balls of your feet. Try standing with your knees locked and feel how your weight automatically shifts to the rear of your feet. Unlock them and feel how your weight automatically shifts toward the front of your feet.

When your knees are softened properly, the sponginess inside will feel somewhat like hard-boiled eggs (sans shell), or like a hard rubber ball, able to flex and give. If your knees are locked, they'll feel sort of like a piece of wood, not able to flex or bend much. When you complete pushoff (where your toes are leaving the ground), that's as close to being straight-legged as you should ever get, and even then it's just for a split second.

Note: If you habitually lock your knees, unlocking them can be difficult because the muscles you need for support may have grown weak through disuse. Take this "softening of the knees" slowly as your muscles get back into shape. The associated exercises will help immensely.

Supportive Gait corrections: 3.2 and 6.1
Strengthening exercises: Semistraight Leg Raises, Modified Mini-
    Squats, Knee Extensions, Groucho Marx
Stretching exercises: Hip Flexor Stretch, Calf Stretch

3.2. Point your knees slightly to the outside. People who lean back often point their knees too far out or too far in. Your leg grows out of your hip at a slight diagonal, which causes your knee, and your foot, to fall open a little naturally. It may seem odd, but when your knees point too far out or too far in the same result occurs—locked knees.

Imagine that your knees are headlights and that you want their beams to light just to the outside of the road ahead. Stand and point in and then out with your knees as headlights, and after the giggling subsides, notice how you can adjust those beams *without* moving your feet. This is important. You don't want to change the *slight* herringbone position of your feet to affect the directional aim of your headlight knees. You actually use a muscle in your hips (the one mentioned in reference to foot pronation, called your sartorius muscle) to turn out those knees. You may feel some muscle tension in your buns, too.

It's possible to have only one knee that doesn't point in the right direction, which usually indicates that your hip muscle (the one that controls that knee) is weaker. It might even hurt when you try to use muscles that have been on vacation until now. Practice with both anyway, and eventually any discomfort or pain should subside as your muscles rebuild.

Although foot and ankle strength are factors in pronation, a weak sartorius muscle is the most common factor. The sartorius is a long, narrow thigh muscle that runs across the front of the thigh from the top of your hip (on the front where you can feel it protrude), to the inside of your tibia (the top of your inner calf). Try feeling that muscle work as you practice depronating. Even when you're standing, if you put your weight toward the outsides of your feet, that act is depronating your feet. To do it, you are using your sartorius muscle.

Supportive Gait corrections: 3.1

Strengthening exercises: Knee/Toe, Standing Sartorius, Half-moons, Semistraight Leg Raises, Slo-Mo Walking (with emphasis on open knees)

Stretching exercises: Wall Stretch Routine, Sitting Stretch Routine

4. Hips

4.1. Increase the width of your step by widening the distance between your feet as you walk. Bowling pins have a narrow base of support because they're designed to fall over. If they had a wide base of support, they'd just scoot off the edge of the alley instead of tipping over. So it's good that bowling pins fall over. Unfortunately, your base of support may be too narrow, like that of a bowling pin. If so, your body is forced to find another, less healthy, means of balancing—hip sitting and leaning back. That means you need to widen your stance.

The word *widen* is one of the most commonly used words at my clinic. When your stance is widened, it invites your body to use the proper muscles to hold you up, rather than letting you rest on your joints (sit in your hips). Imagine a line that goes straight down from your nose, through your navel, and to the floor. The inner edge of your feet should be about two or three inches on either side of that midline.

Since body sizes vary, another way to picture the correct distance between your feet is to find the bony protrusions that stick out at the front of your hips. Go straight down from there, and that's about where your feet should be on the ground as you walk. When your feet are nice and stable, you can derive maximum core strength and avoid all sorts of structural aches, problems, and pains.

Supportive Gait corrections: 6.3

Strengthening exercises: Side-Lying Straight Leg Raises and Hip Circles, Groucho Marx (with really wide steps)

Stretching exercises: Wall Stretch Routine, Sitting Stretch Routine

4.2L. Step wider with your left foot and prevent your right hip from jutting out when you walk. Your right hip is higher than your left, so your body is a bit out of balance. You need to widen your left foot farther to the left by about two extra inches, or until your hips appear to be level (use a mirror). That will reduce the stress on your right side (you've assigned your right side the job of bearing more weight than its share). Stepping out a little wider with your left foot will bring down your right hip so that your pelvis levels, moving all your associated musculature into balance.

If your right hip protrudes when you walk, you're probably leaning back or placing a disproportionate amount of weight on one side. The way to fix that is to pretend there's a waist-high wall directly to your right. Imagine that you're walking close to that wall, almost brushing against it. Visualize that wall so that it blocks your hip from going out with each step. That will help shift your weight back into alignment. If you have trouble with the wall concept, you can substitute an imaginary rope around your hips, lassoed tight, pulling your right hip in just as it starts to jut out. Use a mirror to check your progress.

Strengthening exercises: Inner Thighs, Side-Lying Straight Leg Raises and Hip Circles

Stretching exercises: Wall Stretch Routine, Hip Slider Reaches (hand
  on right hip)

**4.2R. Step wider with your right foot and prevent your left hip
from jutting out when you walk.** Your left hip is higher than your
right, so your body is a bit out of balance. You need to widen your
right foot farther to the right by about two extra inches or until your
hips appear to be level (use a mirror). That will reduce the stress on
your left side (you've assigned your left side the job of bearing more
weight than its share). Stepping out a little wider with your right foot
will bring down your left hip so that your pelvis levels, moving all
your associated musculature into balance.

If your left hip protrudes when you walk, you're probably leaning
back or placing a disproportionate amount of weight on one side.
The way to fix that is to pretend there's a waist-high wall directly to
your left. Imagine that you're walking close to that wall, almost
brushing against it. Visualize that wall so that it blocks your hip from
going out with each step. That will help shift your weight back into
alignment. If you have trouble with the wall concept, you can substitute an imaginary rope around your hips, lassoed tight, pulling your
left hip in just as it starts to jut out. Use a mirror to check your
progress.

Strengthening exercises: Inner Thighs, Side-Lying Straight Leg
  Raises, and Hip Circles
Stretching exercises: Wall Stretch Routine, Hip Slider Reaches (hand
  on left hip)

**4.3. Take longer steps and equalize your stride length on both
sides.** To make sure your steps are longer, you need to increase the
power of your pushoff. As you propel your body forward, make sure
that you really dig in with your big and middle toes and use your bun
muscles on the same side. You should actually feel your bun tighten
with each step. As your bun contracts, allow your weight to move to
the front of that hip just prior to picking up your trailing foot.

So how long should your stride be? One and a half of the length of your feet is the minimum distance your feet should be separated as you walk, measuring from the toes of the back foot to the heel of the front foot. It's just a quick rule of thumb because leg length and other factors come into play, but most people who lean back take short, quick steps. They tend to crash to each next step.

People who lean back also tend to have very little pushoff. Because of this, they also have underdeveloped calf muscles. And they don't have much going for them in the derriere or hamstring department, either, because they underuse both. This results in an exaggerated heel strike, or "heel punch," which pops their feet off the floor and mechanically propels them on to their next step. To fix this, stride with a slightly longer step than normal (remember to lean forward with it). Or incorporate the scissors concept described earlier (imagine a sideview of your legs as scissors, and make the back leg pull back further as your front leg stretches forward). Both techniques extend the use of your buns and hamstrings for a healthier gait.

Note: If one of your steps is not as long as the other, as is often the case when an injury forces you to favor a bad side, try to equalize the length of each step. This should be accomplished by making your shorter step longer, matching the length of the longer stride.

Supportive Gait corrections: 1.3 and 2.2
Strengthening exercises: Standing Hip Flexors, Hip Extensions, Tip-
   toes, Standing Hamstrings, Groucho Marx (with really long steps)
Stretching exercises: Hip Flexor Stretch

4.4. Lengthen the duration of your swing phase. Once again, remember that the swing phase is everything that happens between the time that your toes go airborne until the heel of your same foot strikes the ground again. To establish (or increase) balance, lengthen the duration of your swing phase.

To do that, change the rhythm of your gait so that the swing phase takes just a split second longer. There are different ways to facilitate this. You can slow down your swing phase by adding a "kick step" to your walk, which is when you actually scuff your heel lightly on the floor as your foot moves forward. You'll want to stop scuffing after you've learned to extend the duration of your swing phase. Some people find it easier to accomplish this kick step technique by humming a waltz, or counting in their heads as they "kick-step, kick-step, kick-step."

As you lengthen the duration of your swing, your body is forced to maintain balance by using muscles at the core of your body rather than by falling back on the structural design of your joints and bones. When you balance on your stance phase leg for an extra split second, it forces your abdomen and lower back muscles to hold you up and keep your body in balance. Using those muscles strengthens and sta-bilizes your body to prevent vulnerability and injury.

The body balancing that you accomplish during the swing phase is integral to this entire system of gait corrections because it's what builds the muscles you need to strengthen your powerful "sandwich system." That's the power plant at the core of your body. The sand-wich system is the stabilizing strength of your musculoskeletal pos-ture, particularly the stomach and back muscles, squeezing together at the middle of your torso. It's absolutely essential to the structural stability of your entire spine.

At the other end of the stability spectrum, leaning back causes all the muscles you need for structural balance to grow weak. When those muscles are weak, you tend to lean back even more because it's easier, thus creating an abysmally vicious cycle of structural weakness.

Note: When people lengthen their steps, sometimes they tend to lean back even more as a defensive reaction to the fear of falling. When you lengthen your step you need to be extra vigilant about staying forward, which is covered in Gait Correction 6.1.

Supportive Gait corrections: 1.3, 2.2, 4.3, and 6.1
Strengthening exercises: Hands and Knees Balance, Slo-Mo Walking, Standing Balance
Stretching exercises: Supine Stretch Routine, Hip Flexor Stretch

5. Lower Torso

5.1. Slide your weight from one hip to the other with each step.
Some people who lean back tend to barely shift their weight across
from one hip to the other when they walk. When you neglect that
necessary shift, the result is that too much weight goes crunching
straight into your spine. Properly shifting your weight (with your
middle held tight—using the sandwich system) helps disburse the
load smoothly and evenly throughout your torso.

To shift your weight properly, repeat these words as you walk:
"Step, slide, step, slide." As you say it, do it. Step and then slide
your weight onto that hip. (Be careful not to slide too far, like
many models do for effect. That hip jutting out is just as structurally unsound as not shifting at all. In fact, it has a gait correction all its own.)

In many cases, incorrect weighting can be traced to an injury
(however, that injury may be so old you don't even remember it, and
its ramifications may be barely discernible or totally hidden). When
you injure a joint or muscle, your reflex may be to adjust your weighting to avoid pain on that side. In doing so, you insert (albeit uncon-
sciously) a bad habit into your movement pattern that can generate
structural weakness elsewhere. It may feel normal now, but those
comfort zones are often more insidious than the original injuries.
Asymmetries put undue stress on otherwise perfectly good body
parts.

A patient of mine named Alicia developed an involuntary
reflex shift in weighting where she *lifted* the painful hip, thrust it
forward, and *then* put her foot down. She didn't remember hurting
her hip or leg, but her mini-lurch with that hip indicated
otherwise. The correct way is quite the opposite. Your foot should
step down and *then* your weight should slide over into that hip:
"Step, slide." Alicia also developed what I call a "hip splint" (like
a shin splint, but pain runs along the top boney protuberance of
the hip), which she got rid of when she learned to step and then
slide.

This type of incorrect weighting causes the quadratus lumborum muscle to become tight, which can lead to spasms and pain. How does it become tight? Soft tissue (muscles, tendons, and ligaments) adaptively lengthens when stretched a lot and adaptively shortens when contracted a lot (versus normal momentary lengthening and shortening). Your soft tissue takes on new shapes based on usage as it adapts to these novel positions and movement patterns. So even after the pain has gone, you may still hang on to an old comfort zone pattern based on some reshaping that's taken place. Rebalancing may require going through an uncomfortable period as your muscles, tendons, and ligaments become reshaped to their proper sizes and position.

Note: You may wonder how to ignore the pain and avoid that reflex shift next time you suffer a minor hip strain while jogging, for instance. When that happens to me, which it does (usually to my right hip), I make sure that I open my right knee, widen my stance, and make sure I push into both hips evenly. By doing so I can prevent the pain from expanding beyond a flicker. Once you understand the fundamentals contained in this book, you will develop your own formulas for similar pain prevention and removal. In other words, once you are tuned into your body, you'll notice and fix trouble areas before they become major pains.

Supportive Gait corrections: 6.3
Strengthening exercises: Inner Thighs, Half-moons
Stretching exercises: Hip Slider Reaches (both sides), Supine Stretch Routine (especially the exercises at the end of this stretch routine)

5.2. Don't flatten your spine for "good posture," and please untuck your buns. Some people have been taught to think that the less their buns show, the more attractive their bodies look. These people flatten their spines and tuck their buns under to hide them. But if you work your bun muscles as you walk, you'll replace your plump, tucked-under buns with a tight, well-shaped derriere that you'll be proud to declare. The bottom line is that tucking your buns under is counterproductive to a healthy gait, as well as to a pretty shape. In addition, a lot of people think that a flat spine is good for you. It's not. The tucked-under buns and the flat spine are conjunctive maladies.

In the late 1960s, people with back pain gravitated toward a widely accepted program called the Williams Flexion Exercises. These exercises, done lying down, gained popularity and eventually became incorporated into the way many people walk. What they erroneously concluded was that, if tucking their buns under and lifting up the front of their pelvises was good as an exercise, it must be good for walking, too. Oops, not so.

Some doctors and physical therapists still believe that this is a good way to eliminate back pain. And while the Williams Flexion system certainly has redeeming value, it's still misinterpreted by many professionals and taught *without* the proper focus on strengthening the abs and lower back muscles, which is what this exercise is supposed to be all about.

Recognizing this, a man named Dr. Robin McKenzie entered the spine therapy world. He referred to the victims who misapplied the Williams exercise as "flexion monsters" (people who seemed perpetually stuck in that bun-tucked, straight-spined position). Dr. McKenzie revolutionized the world of back care. He opened the door to a new generation of back-treatment concepts.

Walking with your buns tucked under does not strengthen your belly, as you might expect. Instead, it leads to weak lower abs. These folks need to do trunk flexion *and* extension. Since a strong midsection is absolutely vital to a healthy Primary Movement Pattern, it works to your benefit to untuck your buns, let your spine take on its natural curve, and allow your abs and lower back muscles to work together and grow strong again.

Dr. McKenzie asserted that *backward* movement (in the form of stretching and exercises) was just as important as *forward* movement (the focus of the Williams Flexion Exercises) in reducing back pain. Forward flexion (any movement that brings your nose closer to your knees) is important in the treatment of back pain, but backward flexion (bending back the other way, called back extension) is equally important to the process of restoring muscle strength and spine flexibility. They are both normal spinal movements.

Supportive corrections: 4.3, 5.3, and 6.1
Strengthening exercises: Belly Press, Cross Crawl, Opposite Arm and Leg, Hands and Knees Balance, Hip Extensions
Stretching exercises: Press-Ups, Standing Back Bends, Hip Flexor Stretch

Note: Trunk flexion and extension require lower ab strength. Without ab strength, back exercises can be hard on your spine. So it's best if ab work is done concurrently with your back-extension work. If you have leg pain, you should do the ab exercises only after the leg pain has subsided, otherwise your leg pain may increase. Sometimes doing a few press-ups will reduce the pain right away.

5.3. Hold your belly in (keep it away from your T-shirt). The way to hold your belly in is to imagine trying to keep it from touching your shirt. Attempt to do that all the time. People are often surprised to hear that they have to hold their bellies in. "You mean I have to actually hold it in all the time?" Not when you're sleeping.

Eventually it will become a good habit. It goes hand in hand with bringing your body up and over where it belongs. Both your buns and your belly will almost magically shift toward their proper positions when you're up and over. But this T-shirt trick will help activate your midsection muscles even more.

Strengthening exercises: Alternating Knees, Double Knee to Toes, Table Exercise, Low Ab Knee Switchers

6. Upper Torso

6.1. Bring your upper body "up and over" with a forward cant and your weight on the balls of your feet. Work on bringing your center of gravity forward. To accomplish this most efficiently, tighten your belly muscles a little and make sure that your weight is on the balls of your feet. If you lean back, your center of gravity might be anywhere from your heels to even several inches behind your heels. It should be at the front of your feet or even a few inches out in front of your toes as you walk. Bring your ribs down, tucking them in toward the abdomen cavity, as opposed to splaying your ribs wide and holding them up (see Gait Correction 6.2).

The prototypical example of "good posture" is often exemplified by military men, ballet dancers, models, and good little children who sit up straight. That's a universal misconception, my friends. That "posture" works against your body. When your rib cage is lifted up and widened in the front, or when your chest is raised even a little, it automatically throws your body's weight to the rear, which starts all the problems associated with leaning back.

Here's a little gimmick to help you properly slant (or cant) your whole body forward, bringing your weight onto the balls of your feet. When you walk, imagine that you're heading into a snowstorm, with a formidable wind blowing directly at you. The forward lean you use to compensate for the wind is the action you're looking for. Your body should lean into the wind by bending at the ankles and *without bending over at the waist.*

When I first tell my patients to "cant their bodies forward," I often get some pretty weird contortions. Many people bend at the hips, which not only looks funny but fails to shift their centers of gravity forward. Canting your entire body toward the front starts at the ankles. Picture an Olympic diver (see illustration 5-4) as she's about to dive, perched slightly on the balls of her feet, ready to spring,

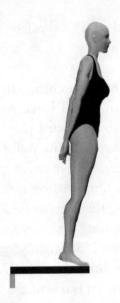

5–4 Correct body position exemplified by diver, with weight on balls of feet, canted slightly forward

appearing to lift up with just the right amount of forward lean. That's the cant you should visualize as you walk.

Here is a test to determine if you're forward enough. Stand your old way, which is probably with your weight on your heels. Drop your chin onto your chest and look down. Do you see any toes down there? Unless you're really slender, you probably see your stomach, or chest, or maybe you can see all the way down to the tips of your shoes. What you should see when you're properly canted forward are the bows of your shoelaces (if your shoes don't have laces, play along). Stand so you can see the bows of your shoelaces. Feel and remember that position. Then get into the habit of assuming that position with every step you take.

Please do not try to look for your shoelaces while you're walking. That would cause your head to tilt down, forcing you to lean back when you walk, thus defeating the entire purpose of this exercise (you will understand this more when you get to the corrections dealing with your head, later in this chapter). You must do this shoelace test while standing, not walking. The shoelace test is only for "feeling" what forward cant is all about.

Note: For every 5 degrees you change the tilt of your body, your keenly acute sense of balance will make you feel like it's tilting 15 degrees. So if you shift your forward plane 15 degrees, it will feel more like 45 degrees, and you'll think you're about to fall forward. If you do, that's a fair indication that you're getting it right. It's awkward at first because your ultrasensitive inner ear and balancing system have got you believing that leaning back is really straight up and down. Your former gait, resting back in your hip joints, isn't vertical, it's actually leaning backward. So when you get vertical, your sensation will be that of falling forward a little. Don't fight it. Look for it. That feeling of falling forward is one of the tools you'll need to walk yourself well.

Supportive Gait corrections: Every correction in this chapter helps with the all-important goal of staying up and over on the balls of your feet. Each correction is interwoven with the rest to produce a fabric of balanced motion.

Strengthening exercises: Belly Press, Cross Crawl, Table Exercise, Double Knees to Toes, Oblique Crunches, Upper Ab Crunches, Low Ab Knee Switchers

Stretching exercises: Supine Stretch Routine, Wall Stretch Routine

6.2. Breathe sideways. This may sound odd, but when you inhale, your ribs should widen as if you're trying to make your lungs and ribs reach for your inner arms. When you exhale, your lungs and ribs should narrow as your belly tightens slightly.

Very often, people who lean back breathe either high up into their chests or into their bellies, both of which throw their bodies up and back. Since the most important objective of this entire system is to keep your weight forward, you don't want a breathing pattern that forces your body toward the rear.

Yoga teachers often tell students to breathe into the belly. I believe that yoga is an exquisite form of meditation and exercise, so I am not going to challenge the ancient traditions of its breathing art. But it's important to know that while breathing into the belly is okay for yoga, it's not okay for walking. You'll need to retrain yourself to breathe sideways when you walk.

We've mentioned some popular misconceptions regarding posture in connection with the military, ballet, and anybody who thinks that holding his or her chin up and breathing into the chest is good. It's not. As you watch trained athletes, you will notice that they pursue a sideways breathing pattern. The chest comes up very little, if at all, and if it does, it comes up at the very end of the breath. Athletes who breathe starting at the top, with their chests up first, are more likely to develop endurance or performance problems than those who breathe more efficiently (sideways).

Sideways breathing is also very important in sitting posture. People who lean back often try to sit up too straight, with their chests up high and their necks and backs strained, breathing straight into the top lobes of their lungs (you have three lobes in your lungs: top, middle, and bottom). Although it's important to use all of them, it is also important to know how to move air into specific lobes by choice. It's easier than you think. (You'll learn more about sitting with structural strength later in "Body Living Lessons," chapter 8.)

Supportive Gait correction: 6.1
Strengthening exercises: Belly Press with Sideways Breathing

6.3. Twist your body when you walk. Rotate your shoulders and turn them toward opposing corners of the room with each step. Your shoulders should not face straight forward as you walk, nor should they move vertically up and down. Instead, the plane of your shoulders should face the corners of an imaginary room as you walk and twist horizontally. Pretend you are walking down the middle of a big room with a ruler straight across your chest so the ends of the ruler are at each shoulder. With each step, turn the ruler on your shoulders toward the corner of the room closest to your leading leg.

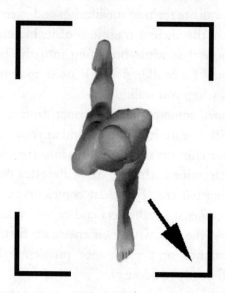

5–5 Correct shoulder rotation facing imaginary corner of room

At the same time that your shoulders face the forward leg (and that corner of the room), your hips will automatically face the other corner. The pivot point of your rotation is in your solar plexus (right below the ribs, in the pit of your stomach). That's where your two halves meet, and that's the axis of your trunk rotation. Your spine runs down your body from the top of your neck to your tailbone, and it should twist in the middle so the bottom half (and everything connected below it) turns one way, while the other half (and everything above it) turns the opposite way. That's how your spine should work when you walk, and it's how you maintain balance—by twisting.

Some people unknowingly attempt to accomplish this twisting action by moving their shoulders without twisting at the solar plexus. They end up looking as if the outer shell is initiating the twist. Movie robots walk like that. And it's not efficient in terms of spinal flexibility, mechanical fluidity, or trunk stability, all of which are necessary to create the diagonal coordination of the four quadrants (your two shoulders and two hips). Still other people attempt to accomplish the twist by throwing their arms, an even less efficient method.

If necessary, reread the information on rotation, including the ice-skater analogy, in chapter 3 (page 43). It's important to grasp the concept of how your torso twists so that your inner core is powering the outer shell. If you don't feel this right away, know that this one takes time to feel. Keep in mind that you can bend your arm loosely, like limp spaghetti, or you can bend it with tension, like you're squeezing a barbell. Both forms of arm tension are initiated and controlled by your mind as you decide which tension to apply. That's the kind of control you can exert throughout your entire body. It's just a matter of getting used to a new level of control over what's going on inside you.

If you think of a line connecting your left hip to your right shoulder, and another line connecting your right hip to your left shoulder, you'd have the shape of an *X*. The middle of the *X* is where the rotation takes place for virtually every forward motion you make, no matter how slight. Take throwing a ball. When both winding up and throwing, notice the diagonal patterns (left and right hips and shoulders). It's the same in all body movement and in virtually every sport (see illustration 5–6).

Eating, swimming, and walking all incorporate the four quadrants of the body, with the two shoulders and two hips as the corners, all working as if they were communicating perfectly with the others. In fact, they are. Body movement, and how the parts interact, is never random. Muscles don't work one at a time; they work in groups. The groups always create diagonal patterns, which create working triangles of movement. Remember that walking is a diagonal, whole-body sport.

One last note about trunk rotation and leaning back. The rotation cannot be done while you're sitting back in your hips. People who lean back have little or no trunk rotation and do not walk with balance.

When teaching rotation, it's easy to spot lapses back to old ways, especially leaning back, because the twist automatically disappears. Conversely, when you successfully integrate other gait corrections, such as positioning yourself up and over, opening your knees, or correcting foot placement, the rotation often comes naturally. So for some people it's easier just to allow the rotation to occur on its own as

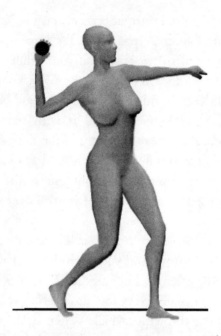

5–6 Natural diagonal patterns of human motion and resulting angle patterns. Notice how many triangles you can locate in this body. Each one is created by a diagonal movement pattern.

the result of some other gait correction. Please be aware of the rotation as it takes place.

Supportive Gait corrections: 3.2, 4.1, 5.1, 6.1, 6.2, and 7.3
Strengthening exercises: Oblique Crunches, Slo-Mo Walking (focus on exaggerating the twist)
Stretching exercises: Clock Stretch

6.4. Pull your chest, shoulders, and back down, and keep your shoulder rotation horizontal. When walking, twist one shoulder forward and the other back—horizontally, not up and down vertically. Softly pull your chest, shoulders, and back down slightly as you walk, and keep your shoulders level.

To get a visual image of how to pull down, imagine a triangle that's upside down and whose three points connect your two shoulders and your belly button. Inside the triangle are bones and muscles that become more efficient when you pull your shoulders down compactly toward the point of the triangle (your navel). At the same time, your shoulder blades should pull down toward your tailbone. Be careful not to round your shoulders while doing this.

One of my worst back patients ever (his back gave him long-term agony) simply could not pull his shoulders down correctly. He carried his arms around like they were crooked baguettes; plus, his shoulders were up so high he looked like he was being carried around on a coat hanger. I'd explain that he needed to pull his shoulders down. He'd try. But he couldn't work it into his new gait. He unintentionally lifted his body up like that as a reflexive response to avoid pain, but it had quite the opposite effect.

He finally made a huge pain-reducing breakthrough as the result of a little trick aimed at keeping his shoulders down. With each step, I asked him to softly brush his thighs with his hands as low as possible without bending over. That worked perfectly for him.

Another trick is to conceptualize growing your arms longer as you walk. Reach for the floor with your middle finger without bringing your shoulders forward, just down. Don't forget, this downward pull on the shoulders happens simultaneously with shoulder rotation as described in Gait Correction 6.3, above. If you're slouching with your shoulders, you've taken the downward pull too far.

Note: If you have pain somewhere between your neck and one shoulder blade, or between your hip and your back on one side, it may be because one shoulder drops and moves in toward your spine as you walk. You should pull your shoulders down softly (but not so they go in toward your spine). If only one of your shoulders tends to pull in that direction when that same arm swings back, try this: at the instant when that arm goes back, reach forward and down a little with your other arm (the forward one). That pulls the deviating arm and shoulder back up a bit. If both shoulders bob up and down, refer to Gait Correction 6.3.

Supportive Gait corrections: 6.2, 6.3, 7.2, 7.4, and 8

Strengthening exercises: Modified Push-ups, Scapular Push-ups, Sitting Lats, Slo-Mo Walking, Back Shoulder Rolls

Stretching exercises: Clock Stretch

7. Arms

7.1. Use your arms, don't carry them. Feel your arms and *use* them as you walk. Experience the muscles and the movement. With your thumbs forward and your pinkies to the rear, follow through with your arms using the momentum generated at your solar plexus (the center of your body, where the twist begins).

Your arms should feel slight tension all the way down to your fingertips. Although they're moving forward and back like a pendulum, your arms are not meant to swing like dead weight or be carried like tubes of liverwurst. They're tools that should assist in the process of propelling your body forward.

Strengthening exercises: Cross Crawl, Modified Push-ups, Scapular Push-ups, Sitting Lats, Opposite Arm and Leg, Slo-Mo Walking

Stretching exercises: Pec Stretch in a Doorjamb

7.2. Increase or decrease the angles of your arm swing. The distance your arm travels to the front should be the same as the distance it travels to the rear. People who lean back tend to have a bigger arm swing backward than forward, and they are usually unaware of it. Even when your weight is properly forward, sometimes its easy to swing too far forward (especially while you're first learning).

Because swinging your arms is such a reflexive action, thinking about how far your arms should go can make you crazy. Don't stress. Just keep in mind that proper arm swing is rather small—about 15 to 20 degrees.

Strengthening exercises: Slo-Mo Walking, Modified Push-ups, Scapular Push-ups, Sitting Lats

Stretching exercises: Seated Back and Neck Stretch, Shoulder Rolls

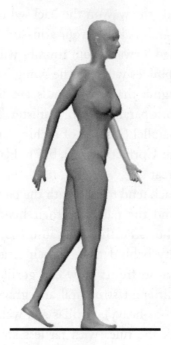

5–7 Correct arm swing

7.3. Move your arms straight through, not around the body. People who lean back frequently let their arms swing out away from their bodies as if they're centrifugal appendages. That's counterproductive. Move your arms in a straight line, forward and back.

Imagine that each of your middle fingers has a pencil taped on to it so that each arm swing draws a line that marks the movement of your hands. From a top view looking down, the lines should be straight—like this: ||; not like parentheses: ().

Strengthening exercises: Scapular Push-ups, Sitting Lats, Slo-Mo
    Walking
Stretching exercises: Seated Back and Neck Stretch, Shoulder Rolls

7.4. Let your thumbs lead the way to the front. Your thumbs should be the most forward part of your hand as you swing your arm forward. Your pinky leads the way on the backswing. Since your shoulder is basically a ball and socket, if your arms are on straight and your shoulders are not rolled forward, your thumbs will naturally lead your arm swing and your pinkies will lead the swing backward.

As you walk, imagine that your hands are lightly grasping and gliding along a smooth parallel bar or banister. This not only keeps your arms running parallel (instead of arching around the body like parentheses—see Gait Correction 7.3), but holds your thumbs to the front, pinkies to the rear.

People who lean back tend to lead with the backs of their hands on the forward swing and the palms of their hands on the backward swing. Gorillas do the same thing because they, too, tend to carry their center of gravity behind them. Their heads are forward and their arms hang down in front. How can gorillas get away with it? Aside from having different structural and gravitational issues than humans (they're bottom-heavy), gorillas are, well, as strong as gorillas, so they can break the rules with far less structural vulnerability than humans. And who knows, maybe they have back pain and just aren't telling us.

Strengthening exercises: Modified Push-ups, Scapular Push-ups, Sitting Lats, Back Shoulder Rolls

Stretching exercises: Pec Stretch in a Doorjamb, Clock Stretch, Seated Back and Neck with Shoulder Rolls

8. Head

8.1. Keep your head up and back. Bring your chin and your eyes down slightly. People who lean back almost always have their heads too far forward. Because of that, it's easy to spot a person who is a candidate for back pain. When they sit or walk, it looks like they're being gently pulled by the nose. Instead, keep your head up and back, above your torso, not out in front of you leading the way.

It's often unnecessary to address the subject of head position if everything else is in balance. Given some time, your head tends to right itself when your torso is where it should be, over your hips and not behind them. When your torso is in place, your head will not stick out in front.

Athletes look in the direction they want to go not just because they fear crashing into things but because human motion naturally follows the line of sight. Your eyes direct your head, and your head directs your body.

In the case of walking, your focus (and the direction of your head) should be on the ground, usually about twenty to twenty-five feet in front of you. Your chin and your eyes should be tilted slightly downward, exposing the crown of your head to your approaching admirers. People who lean back tend to have their heads forward, and only their eye sockets look down. When your head is tilted at the proper angle, your eyes will focus twenty to twenty-five feet ahead without any eyeball movement. (Some people keep their heads up and their chins out just to keep their glasses from falling off. Loose glasses are a strange yet common reason for tumultuous years of back pain.)

Many patients grasp other aspects of a proper gait, only to surrender to this last urge to keep their chin up. Maybe you hold your chin high as part of your personality, or to project confidence, or to show when you're emphatic, which makes it even harder to let go. As soon as your chin and eyes go up, you tend to raise your chest, slide into your hips, and once again lean back when you walk. For other patients, the opposite holds true. No matter what their success is with the other gait corrections, as soon as they lower their chin, their weight shifts forward automatically. Once they understand the system, this one correction often makes the other corrections fall right into place.

Either way, learn to feel and analyze the position of your head so that it remains your body's favorite passenger.

Supportive Gait correction: 6.4
Strengthening exercises: Neck Diagonals, Neck Flexors, Neck Extensions, Side-Lying Neck Rotations
Stretching exercises: Seated Back and Neck Stretch, Shoulder Rolls, Clock Stretch

LEARNING THE SPORT OF WALKING

In the beginning, you'll feel like you're made of a bunch of parts that don't know how to work together anymore. It's like going back to square one on something you thought you'd learned when diapers still fit you. Then you'll add a new gait correction, only to find that you lost the one you thought you'd just perfected. Then your best friend will snigger or tell you that you're walking "weird." These tribulations are to be expected.

Respond with a higher level of resolve. Generate the tenacity to forge ahead one small step at a time. Let yourself relax between sessions, letting go of the whole thing. The small, concentrated units of practice will take you where you want to go.

After a while, you'll focus on a particular correction and the others you've learned will naturally be summoned into action. It's like learning a new sport, or taking piano lessons, only not as hard. The similarities lie in the need to relax and persevere.

Finally you'll get it. You'll see yourself doing all these things naturally. You'll be walking down the sidewalk and catch a glimpse of yourself, maybe see a reflection in a storefront window, and you'll recognize what a beautiful gait you have—strong, confident, and best of all, one that will let you eliminate or prevent structural pain.

≋ 6 ≋

STRENGTHENING EXERCISES

EXERCISES THAT CORRESPOND TO YOUR GAIT CORRECTIONS

Almost every gait correction has a few exercises to go with it. These exercises significantly augment your new primary movement strategy by strengthening areas of your body that might have become weak through disuse. When those muscles get stronger, it gets easier to adjust to your new gait.

Some exercises have the added benefit of incorporating movement patterns that emulate those required for a balanced gait. In addition to strengthening beneficial muscle groups, they familiarize you (and your body) with structurally sound walking patterns. On top of all the structural benefits you'll derive, an added bonus comes your way in the form of cosmetic value. These exercises are guaranteed to tighten and tone various parts of your body. You're going to look as great as you feel.

Unlike your gait correction routine, which consists of at least four short practice sessions spread out evenly during the day, these exercises can be done anytime and without any special regularity. It will be more effective if you do your exercises at least every other day to promote the changes you want. And if you're really driven to achieve the maximum results in the shortest amount of time, you can do more. Just add on slowly and adjust as you check yourself constantly for pain relief, new or intensified pain, fatigue, and how the corrections and exercises are working for you.

Rather than pick the exercises for you, I've listed all the possibilities. Some will work better than others, and it's totally acceptable to choose only the exercises that you've found work best for you.

STRENGTHENING BY-LAWS

As for specific rules governing exercise, it's virtually impossible to come up with a set of one-size-fits-all parameters. However, there are a few by-laws that apply to everyone, and they'll help you create your own personal program of strengthening.

You Own It . . . Feel It!

Tune in to your body. Know what it feels like when a particular muscle is at work. Don't wait until you've strained a muscle to notice it. Increase your awareness of what's happening inside of you now.

Many people with keen minds for finance, software programming, and even medicine, are sometimes just too busy to step up the intensity with which they know their bodies. They may take the body for granted and neglect treating it like the precision instrument it really is. Your body can benefit from more than just fuel and minor maintenance, especially if you expect pain-free operation.

In conjunction with this book, you can turn up your level of awareness and recognize the control you have over your body. Notice how you can completely relax your arm—or vigorously squeeze it like you were gripping a hammer. You can simulate muscle resistance by supplying directions from your mind. Your brain is used to it. You can choose to be aware of the various muscle groups at work as you walk to the kitchen, or just focus on the smell of that coffee (both sound pretty good). You can experience your foot muscles working, or you can let your feet flap around at the ends of your legs unnoticed. You can feel your buns contract as you walk, or you can let them hang anonymously underneath you.

Imagine muscle contractions on a scale of one to ten, where ten is power-on and taut, and one is your basic Jell-O. Some people go on day after day without realizing that the body, and their concept of it, can be more than gelatin. They live at zero all the time. Some people do pay attention to their bodies and just need to be encouraged to learn more. This is your chance to break through to level ten. Feel the interaction of your parts and use those parts to build a Primary Movement Pattern that lets you walk yourself well with every step you take. You get to own the experience.

Repetitions and Weight

Repetitions are the number of cycles you perform during one set of a particular exercise. If you do five sit-ups, take a rest, and do five more, that's two sets of five repetitions (or "reps"). As you observe and learn what your body parts are up to, you also need to learn how to adjust your repetitions in accordance with your own personal limits.

My patients always ask me "How many of this [or that] exercise should I do?" It's not a bad question. Especially if you're in pain and concerned about reinjury. But only *you* can know when you're not working hard enough, when you're putting forth solid effort, and when you're pushing things a bit too far. It may take time. You'll have to stay in touch with every movement at each moment. Keep in mind that new things are hard at first and that relearning things you already thought you knew is even harder. Be patient with yourself. No name-calling.

One of my patients is a wonderful, healthy older woman whom I hope to emulate when I get into *my* late eighties. She golfs all the time, swims in a lap pool, and recently decided to learn how to walk again. She worked diligently and nailed her target. She walked away from old habits like a bad fashion, after eighty years of "already knowing how to walk." When young patients squeak to me that they can't change thirty years of ingrained patterns, I love to tell them about Leona.

Getting back to repetitions and weight, Leona loves to tell me that I don't know a number lower than thirty. True. I start there whenever I can, and it's a pretty good number of reps when divided into three sets of ten. That's average for most everybody. But your weight and proportions should dictate the actual numbers.

If you find that three sets of ten is too much, then try three sets of a lower number. You may start at three sets of five. When you're serious, your last few reps will feel like they're almost too hard to do. After you've done that many for a few days (or if you're being conservative, a few weeks), then go to three sets of four and stay there for a while. Work up to three sets of ten.

When ten reps gets easy, add some weight where applicable, a little at a time. With extremity work, such as lower ab exercises, add one pound on each foot. It will barely feel noticeable. If you don't feel like running out to the store to buy a set of one-pound weights, which you will quickly outgrow anyway, try putting seventy-five pennies (they weigh half a pound) in each of an old pair of socks. Tie the socks together at both ends and hang the resulting "bracelet" on your wrist or ankle. It's more cost-effective and efficient to find a set of weights that can be added to incrementally, like a cuff weight with Velcro that has removable half pounds (they make one- to five-pounders). When you can do one pound thirty times without a problem, add more.

So maybe you're asking "How much strengthening do I need to do, and how do I protect my body from injury along the way?" Good questions. After a back accident and three successful months of therapy, a woman once asked me when she would be done. I recalled that she performed her exercises with precision and proper alignment. She knew the routine. But then I remembered that she could barely get through most of her exercises (thirty reps without weights). Also, as she left my gym and thought I wasn't watching, or perhaps she just wasn't concentrating, her gait would slip into leaning back a little.

(And this woman wanted to become pregnant soon!) She needed more strengthening exercises.

Another patient of mine performed her exercises with similar precision and proper alignment. In two months she was almost up to my level of fitness. (I like to keep my strength up to where I can execute fifty reps with two to three pounds on my feet for all of my hip and ab work.) Though she did not ask me when she would be done with the exercises, she clearly had the system worked into her Primary Movement Pattern and could probably get away with not exercising as much without jeopardizing a thing. That's because she was practicing, strengthening, balancing, and stabilizing every time she walked.

Left and Right Sides

Some of the exercises described in this chapter have two sides to them: a left and a right. It's important to do both sides, even if only one side is particularly tight, uneven, or injured. Doing both sides will help keep your body in balance. There is no reference within the exercise explanations that tells you to do both sides. Semistraight Leg Raises, for example, are explained in terms of how to raise one of your legs. Please remember to do the other one.

About Doing and Overdoing

Overdoing strengthening work is usually less insidious than overdoing stretching work, but here are some guidelines. It's okay to need aspirin for soreness. Nothing bad will happen to you as a result of muscle soreness, within reason. The worst mistakes generally are made when people use too much weight. I once had a patient who decided to get rid of her inner thigh bulge all in one day. Whoa, girl. She couldn't walk without severe thigh pain for two weeks. Needless to say, nothing much in the way of positive results occurred. In fact, she took a giant step backward because she couldn't move without howling and so exercise was out of the question.

When I'm in one of those crazy, driven moods and I want to do more, I add more reps instead of adding more weight. You'll find that the soreness is more manageable and you don't have to miss days or weeks of workouts because you overdid anything. Weight can really only be taken up slowly and systematically. Add a pound at a time. Then feel, observe, and monitor your response to additional reps and weight.

Plan to do big workouts with heavy weights every other day, so as not to bombard your system. But the exercises in this book are not very monstrous, so it's perfectly fine to do them daily. If you're jammed up timewise, then exercise every other day. You'll still get there. Some of my patients divide their exercises into an A day and a B day, and do half of their program on A and the other half on B. That works well for getting things done in smaller increments of time. Doing something is better than doing nothing, so even if you exercise only once or twice a week, you can still accomplish a lot.

Exercise Pain

The key to strengthening is to challenge muscles in a systematic way that forces them to grow stronger. That means it has to be hard. The last few repetitions are supposed to be difficult. Okay, I'm pussyfooting around here. They're supposed to hurt, but it's the type of hurt that you can learn to love—honest.

When you feel you can't do another one, you can. If you allow yourself to be distracted by music or thoughts that remove your attention from the discomfort, you'll find you can do more. I'm talking about a pure kind of muscle soreness, like a bruise or an ache, not the pain that you feel with inflammation due to injury. You'll know the difference because they have two distinct flavors. I find myself asking patients all the time, "Does this pain feel like the original pain you were trying to eliminate when you came in to my office the first time? No? Then do more."

Structural Pain

If you methodically increase your weight and reps but you still have your original pain, you may be up against a structural problem, not muscle soreness. If you suspect the former, you may need to change things a bit. Sometimes you'll work on a part of your body that does not hurt, but the position you have to be in, or the complementary muscles you use, start the original pain all over again. That indicates a structural problem. Watch out for that, especially if it worsens after you've stopped exercising. Experiment by modifying your exercise routine.

Learn to recognize what's transpiring as the result of which movements and what exercises. Then after you've gently stretched, pampered, iced, soothed, soaked, or otherwise healed yourself of that pain, come back to your exercises more slowly, or modify the position to safeguard from further problems. Or just choose another exercise that works for that gait correction.

Every week, at least one patient tells me that he or she used to exercise before his or her injury (whatever the injury was that eventually led the patient into my clinic) but stopped so as not to worsen his or her condition. I don't think I've ever instructed a patient to do nothing. That's counterproductive. There's *always* something to do to keep some part of your body in shape. Pregnant women, stuck in bed, can still do small isometrics or gentle stretches. Of course, if you're healing from a new trauma, there are times when rest is best, but usually it's better to incorporate exercise around an injury. As long as you go slowly, check and recheck, wait for a day or two if necessary, and check again, you can gauge your own tolerances.

Breathing

As a general rule, it's standard to exhale as you exert, or do work, and inhale as you prepare, or relax. When you exhale, push your diaphragm down. This will boost your output level because it engages your abs. Almost every act of strength starts with a stable trunk and some ab tightening. When you exhale and tighten your belly for hip or shoulder extension, you can get through those last few painful reps more easily. Try exhaling during the downward part of your golf swing, or as you lift off the ice for a jump, or as you serve a tennis ball, or as you lift a suitcase (lifting correctly, of course). You'll find that you can accomplish more that way.

At first, breathing correctly may seem like too much to learn. People complain to me all the time about it. Don't feel alone if you hate this part. But after you've done it correctly for a few weeks, you'll never be able to exercise again without using it. Inhale and relax, exhale for the work. With hip, knee, and upper ab work, it's exhale up.

Diet

For muscles to strengthen and grow, you've got to eat protein. Muscle is made of mostly protein. I feel that this whole country has become protein-starved between the vegetarian movement and the high-carbohydrate enthusiasts. If meat, fish, and poultry are not on your list of acceptable foods, you can get protein in other ways. When you eat certain vegetables together, they supply the essential amino acids that make up protein. Tofu has built-in protein, ready to go. And there are zillions of books to help you out with this, but basically, when you're trying to strengthen, I recommend that you eat some protein at every meal.

Go For It!

Here is a list of all the Strengthening Exercises, followed by the page number on which each one is explained.

STRENGTHENING EXERCISES

1. Towel Scrunches

Technical Purpose: To strengthen the arches of your feet.

Gait Application: The primary goal here is to decrease pronation. A balanced gait starts with a solid connection to the floor. Weak arches cause pronation. And ironically, pronation weakens your arches. At mid-stance, when all your weight is on one foot, your arches need to be in good shape to generate stability.

Preparation: Sit with your feet flat, knees at 90 degrees. Put a towel on the ground, outstretched under your feet, extending forward from your heels.

The Exercise: Scrunch your toes under to grab little bits of the towel and pull it toward you, piece by piece, or inch by inch. Pull it by bunching it all up into your arches. If you have trouble scrunching up the towel, it's a little easier if your foot is damp, so a little bowl of

6–1 Towel Scrunches

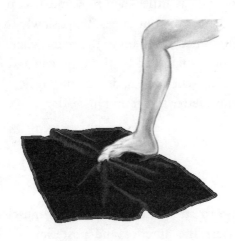

water nearby can be handy for the soles of your feet. One of the mottoes around our clinic is "a towel a day."

2. Alphabet

Technical Purpose: To strengthen, tone, and stretch all the muscles around the ankle, especially the anterior and posterior tibialis, peroneals, gastrox/soleus, and the arch or plantar muscles.

Gait Application: Helps you to hold your toes up longer, depronate your feet, strengthen your arches, and is very useful in reducing shin splints.

Preparation: Sit on something high like a washer, dryer, kitchen counter, or bathroom sink, so your legs can dangle. Sit so you are well supported, not too close to the edge, but close enough so your legs dangle freely. Start with your knees and feet about hip width. Sit up tall and don't slouch, and feel free to use your hands as a brace for balance.

The Exercise: Draw the alphabet, using your big toe like a paintbrush. You can do this with both feet simultaneously or one foot at a time. Really move your ankles around to get that big toe drawing large capital letters with as little knee movement as possible. Your ankles do the work here, not your knees. Start slowly to get familiar with big toe painting. Then speed up to the point where your ankles, feet, and shins are pretty fatigued by the time you're done with the alphabet. The whole alphabet once a day should suffice. If the alphabet gets boring, write a letter to a friend instead.

3. Fish Feet

Technical Purpose: To strengthen the peroneal muscles and ankle dorsiflexors, which are the anterior and posterior tibialis muscles. This exercise also strengthens the arches of your feet.

Gait Application: People who lean back when they walk do so without properly lifting their feet and their toes. As a result, they adeptly avoid an intrinsic element of balanced movement. When you use your feet and toes properly, your swing phase lasts just a split second longer, and that forces you to balance yourself using all of your stabilizing musculature, especially your hips and trunk. That split second of holding your balance epitomizes the strengthening action that should take place with every step (using the sandwich system).

Preparation: Sit on something high like a washer, dryer, kitchen counter, or bathroom sink, so your legs can dangle. Sit so you are well supported, not too close to the edge, but close enough so your legs dangle freely. Put a towel under you so the edge doesn't hurt. Start with your knees and feet about two inches apart. Sit up tall and don't slouch, and feel free to use your hands as a brace for balance.

The Exercise: Roll your feet out as if you are trying to point your inner ankles down toward the floor (but you need to keep your legs hanging down pretty straight). Then bring the bottoms of your feet toward each other like they're kissing or attempting to clap. Remember that this is an ankle exercise, so the less leg movement, and the more ankle movement, the better.

6–3 Fish Feet

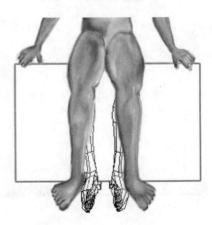

4. Toes Feet/Feet Toes

Technical Purpose: To strengthen the toe lifters (extensors) and the foot lifters (ankle dorsiflexors) in functional sequences that exaggerate what's required of those muscles when you walk. This exercise also strengthens your arches.

Gait Application: People who lean back often have feet that are so underdeveloped they look like cute little pudgy infants' feet. The muscles of a person's feet indicate whether or not they lean back. In general, our feet are grossly neglected and underestimated in terms of their functional potential. I've actually heard of doctors telling their patients that foot problems have nothing to do with their back pain. That scares me. I've also heard doctors say that there's no need to exercise your feet since they're adequately worked just by walking around. The trouble is that they're walking around using the inadequate patterns that caused the problem in the first place. You need to exercise and develop those little muscles. They need to be in prime shape.

The actual gait application is this: at the start of each swing phase, your foot muscles are all working together to lift your toes and feet, which begins the motion that clears your leg off the ground. Folks who lean back don't properly shorten their legs for ground clearance. Instead they usually bounce them off the ground in a

6–4 Toes Feet/Feet Toes

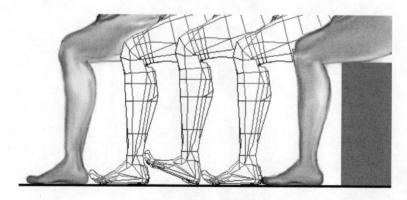

mechanical reflex, and their feet travel through the air like a penguin's, flat and floppy.

The Exercise: Sit on a chair with your feet flat on the floor (knees bent at 90 degrees). Rest your elbows on your knees and lean forward so you can watch your feet and add resistance to the exercise in the form of upper-body weight. Lift your toes first, making sure that your ankles stay neutral (that is, not rolled in or out) and that you lift all five toes if you can. Spread your toes as you lift them and keep the balls of your feet on the ground.

Next, lift your feet farther. This time keep your heels on the ground. Now, put the balls of your feet down while still holding your toes up and spread. (It may be hard to spread your toes at first. But it's easier than a lot of other things you'll be trying for the first time. Just keep on thinking about spreading those toes and they will spread.) Finally, put your toes down. Do fifty or one hundred a day, and in a few weeks you'll be done with this one.

5. Knee Extensions

Technical Purpose: To aggressively strengthen the quadriceps muscles.

Gait Application: Your quadriceps muscles, in combination with your abdominal muscles, are extremely relevant during mid-stance, when all of your weight is on one foot (because the other foot is busy swinging past your leg). Your quads keep your knee from locking or collapsing, just as your abs keep you from falling over (now that you're no longer depending on your hip joints to hold you up).

This exercise is an exaggerated version of those two muscles working together. (Other muscles are at work during this exercise, too!) If you have pain in either of your knees or your back, you can limit the range of this exercise accordingly. Either bend less or straighten less (or both) to limit the range.

Preparation: Sit on something high like a washer, dryer, kitchen counter, or bathroom sink, so your legs can dangle. Sit so you are well supported, not too close to the edge, but close enough so your legs dangle freely. Start with your knees and feet at about hip width and your feet flexed up, not pointing toward the floor. Sit up tall and don't slouch, and feel free to use your hands as a brace. You can even lean up against something for back support, but limit that practice as much as possible (you get a better workout without the back support).

The Exercise: Exhale and raise one or both legs at the same time. It's best to raise both at once because you elicit the complementary help of the abs, but if that feels uncomfortable for any reason, you can strengthen your quads aggressively one at a time. It takes quite a few of these to be effective, whether as single- or double-leg lifts. So if you experienced no negative repercussions from a couple of sets of twenty-five, go ahead and move up to thirty-five, fifty, or more. Start adding weight one pound at a time when it's comfortable to do two sets of fifty. Exhale as you lift, inhale as you lower. Some people

6–5 Knee Extensions

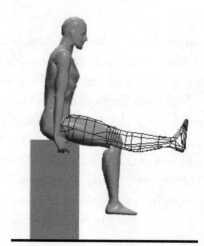

(like me) do fifty to one hundred of these with five pounds on each ankle. I had to work up to that very slowly, too.

6. Semistraight Leg Raises

Technical Purpose: To strengthen the quadriceps muscle for all three parts of the knee (inside, front, and outside). The quads control your knee bend. Some quad exercises are done straight-legged, but this exercise helps strengthen the knee when the legs are in the soft-knee position (slightly bent).

Gait Application: Facilitates staying forward on your feet by strengthening the muscles you need most to walk with springy knees. Remember that when you lock your knees, or fail to walk with them slightly bent and springy, you automatically tend to lean back.

Preparation: Find a chair, or something else to sit on so that when seated your legs are bent at about 90 degrees. Sit forward in the chair so you're on the edge with your back straight and your belly tight. Extend one leg out in front of you and rest your heel on the floor. Bend your knee slightly (people tend to bend too far with this exercise).

6–6 Semistraight Leg Raises

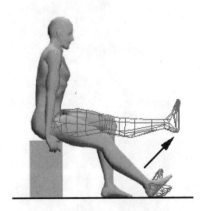

The Exercise: Exhale as you raise your leg (the one with your foot forward) up to the height of the other knee. If you can't lift it that far, that's okay, as long as you're lifting without shifting your back or locking your knee to get your leg up higher. Keep your knee slightly bent and your back straight up and down when you lift. Tilting your back or straightening your knee makes it easier to do but also defeats the purpose of the exercise. Back straight, knee slightly bent.

7. Standing Hamstrings

Technical Purpose: To aggressively strengthen the hamstrings in the standing position. It's really efficient to work on your hamstrings in a standing position because you can add the resistance you need while simultaneously safeguarding your back. At the same time, you exercise your abs (if you stay lifted up and forward).

Gait Application: This exercise combines hamstring development with balance and abdominal strengthening, all of which augment your gait during mid-stance.

6–7 Standing Hamstrings

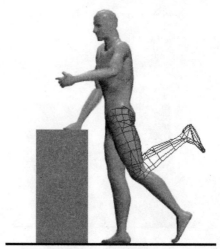

Preparation: Stand with one hand holding on to something at around waist level, like a countertop, and have the other hand outstretched to the side for balance. Move your weight forward onto the ball of your front foot. Keep your chin down, as well as your chest, and put one leg behind you with just your toes touching the floor.

The Exercise: Exhale as you raise your heel toward your buttocks. Inhale as you lower your foot until your toes touch down again. This exercise can be done with no hand support (both arms up), in which case it becomes an even better exercise because it incorporates additional balancing, ab strength, and trunk stabilization with hamstring development.

8. Modified Mini-Squats

Technical Purpose: To strengthen your knees (quads and hamstrings) and to stabilize and strengthen your trunk.

Gait Application: Knee flexion and trunk stabilization are both part

6–8 Modified Mini-Squats

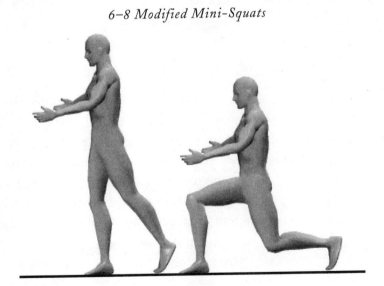

of a healthy gait, and are vital in the balancing act of walking. This exercise is similar to the Groucho Marx but is more strenuous.

Preparation: Stand with one foot about twelve inches in front of the other foot. Put the back foot on its toes while distributing your weight evenly between both feet. On your forward foot, the weight should be at the ball of the foot. Set your shoulders, chest, and chin down, and outstretch both arms slightly in front of your body like you're holding a big beach ball.

The Exercise: Exhale and lower your body. As you lower, hold your belly tight, keep your buns under your torso, and point your chin slightly down. Inhale as you raise your body straight up again. You should go down only as far as is comfortable for your knees. You need to be able to come back up again to a full standing position without losing your balance. In the beginning that may mean you go just a few inches down, a perfectly acceptable start. If you have knee problems, same thing. You should compensate by doing more reps.

Note: For this exercise, starting with three sets of ten per side might be too much. Start with three sets of five per side and see how your quads feel the next day before you add more reps.

9. Dial Outs

Technical Purpose: To strengthen the hip internal rotators. People with too much foot turnout often have leg pain or sciatic pain because too much foot turnout slowly shortens the piriformis muscle, which in turn squeezes down on the sciatic nerve, which runs straight through it. Many patients who have been diagnosed as having a bad disk experience an amazing recovery when they work on stretching their piriformis muscles and strengthening their counterbalancing muscles, the hip internal rotators. By the way, foot turnout is quite common and is not relegated just to dancers.

Gait Application: In Gait Correction 3.2 the goal was to control the direction of your "headlight knees" so that they were turned slightly out. As you develop your new gait, this knee-pointing stuff can be very confusing, especially if your feet turn out to begin with. This exercise will help your internal rotator strength so your hips gain the dexterity to help stabilize your knee.

Preparation: Sit on something high like a washer, dryer, kitchen counter, or bathroom sink, so your legs can dangle. Sit so you are well supported, not too close to the edge, but close enough so your legs dangle freely. Start with your knees and feet at about hip width, and your feet flexed up, not pointing toward the floor.

The Exercise: Exhale as you move both feet straight up and out to the sides while keeping your knees still (your knees should be about six inches apart). Inhale as you move your legs back down. Exhale out, inhale back down. Don't worry if your feet don't go very far to start with. Even with a little bit of movement, you'll get the right effect.

6–9 Dial Outs

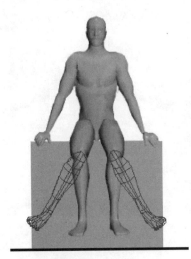

10. Standing Sartorius

Technical Purpose: One of the primary jobs of your sartorius muscle is to support your knee in such a manner that it can stay slightly open as you walk (headlight knees slightly out). If your sartorius muscle is weak, your knee and foot roll in during mid-stance instead of staying open. That makes it very difficult for your hip rotators to remain stable enough to do their job of supporting the spine, which ultimately stabilizes your entire trunk.

Gait Application: The sartorius muscle has two other very important jobs besides holding your knee open. It pulls your knee out, which lifts the ankle away from pronation. It also supports your hips. This exercise stabilizes your hips and helps develop a strong sandwich system.

Preparation: Find something to hold on to for balance and stand next to it sideways. Set your eyes, chin, chest, and ribs slightly down, and stretch out your free arm to the side and a little in front of you, with your elbow slightly bent. Put most of your weight on the foot closest to the hand support. Twist your unweighted leg over and

6–10 Standing Sartorius

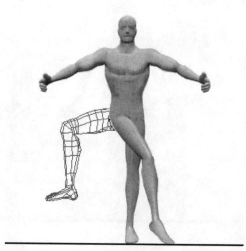

across your other leg like a corkscrew, pointing your toes down and in.

The Exercise: Exhale and pull your knee up and out so that the inside of your knee is facing forward. If you can't get it to face forward all the way, get as close as you can while keeping your hips facing forward. It's a common mistake to allow your hip to pull back, which creates less work for the sartorius and thus diminishes the strengthening effects of this exercise. Inhale and twist your leg back down and in to the first position, over and across your other leg. Repeat, moving from up and out to down, across, and in, and back to up and out. Exhale on the up and out, inhale on the down and in.

11. Side-Lying Straight Leg Raises and Hip Circles

Technical Purpose: Strengthens your gluteus medius and tensor fascia lata, with secondary benefits to your hip adductors and your quadriceps. In other words, this exercise is designed for the outer hip, but other muscles are assisting and receiving secondary benefits.

Gait Application: Strengthens your hips and at the same time builds a strong sandwich system to stabilize your spine. This exercise prepares you for walking with *wide*, stable steps that ultimately lead to staying forward on your feet. This is another exercise that combines strengthening with the actual motions of a correct gait.

Preparation: Lie on the floor on your side (either side) with your bottom leg slightly bent. Your top leg should rest on the bottom leg, but it should be straight (neither bent nor hyperextended—straight). Keep your hips absolutely straight up and down, so a ruler standing upright (perpendicular to the floor) would touch both hipbones at the same spot. Rest on your bottom arm and use your top arm for support, hand in front of you on the floor. Or you can use your bottom arm as a prop, elbow on the floor and hand sort of cupping your head just behind (or on) your ear.

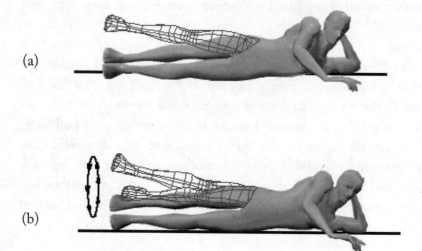

(a)

(b)

6–11 (a) Side-Lying Straight Leg Raises (b) Hip Circles

The Exercise:

Leg Raises: Exhale and tighten your belly as you raise your top leg to shoulder height, but not any higher. Your leg should be straight, foot flexed, and you should imagine that your leg is being stretched longer by the heel, almost like someone is pulling on it. Hold your leg at hip height for a second, and then exhale as you slowly lower your leg down again. If you have a difficult time unlocking your knees, you can do this exercise with your knee slightly bent. Also, be careful not to crash-land your foot to the floor. Control the landing to maximize strengthening. Once you have mastered the Leg Raises, move on to the Hip Circles.

Hip Circles: Exhale, tighten your belly, and simultaneously raise your leg up to shoulder height. While the leg is in the air, make between five and ten small circles about the size of a basketball with your foot (heel extended like it's being stretched longer again), remembering to raise your foot no higher than your shoulder. Draw the circles slowly, inhaling at the bottom of each circle and exhaling as you go up again. Keep the circles small so your body doesn't rock around, and feel your belly tighten to stabilize your midsection (this exercise helps the abs, too). Start slowly to get the feel of the circles, and be careful not to chop off the back half of the circle. Most people tend to cut off the back half because it requires the most strength. Try not to cheat, and make sure your foot is flexed, heel extended away from you. Do an equal number of forward and backward circles.

12. Knee/Toe

Technical Purpose: To strengthen the sartorius muscle as it works in conjunction with your gluteus maximus to pull your hip into extension as you walk.

Gait Application: The sartorius keeps your knee slightly open at heel strike, which helps lift the foot out of pronation. This works in conjunction with the gluteus maximus, which keeps you from falling forward as your weight passes over your hip. This exercise focuses on that part of your gait.

Preparation: Lie on your side. Lean up on your forearm and put your other hand on the floor in front of you for additional support. Make sure you don't collapse into your supporting shoulder (no turtling). Then bend your top leg at the knee and place that foot behind the knee of your front leg. Your bottom leg should be bent a little.

6–12 Knee/Toe

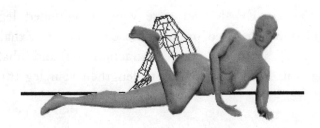

The Exercise: Inhale and bring the knee of your back leg over, rotating your hip as little as possible, and touch that knee to the floor out in front of you. Exhale as you lift your knee back up into the air, bringing your top leg behind you, and touch only your toes to the floor behind the knee of your lower leg. When your knee is pointing up at the ceiling and you take your leg farther back, you can increase the workout on your sartorius and gluteus maximus.

13. Inner Thighs: Top Leg Back and Top Leg Forward

Technical Purpose: To strengthen the long and short adductor muscles (the lower part of the inner thigh and the upper part of the inner thigh).

Gait Application: This exercise helps to develop the muscles that generate the width of your step. Your inner thigh muscles are in charge of that department. If you like jumping (as I do for ice-skating), this is the muscle you need to generate height. Basketball players, this one is for you.

Top Leg Back
Preparation: Lie on your side, but roll your hip back just enough so that your weight is really resting more on your bun. Lean up on your forearm and put your other hand on the floor in front of you for additional support. Don't collapse into your shoulder. Then bend your top leg at the knee and place that foot behind the knee of your other leg. Your bottom leg should be straight, knee turned slightly out, foot flexed.
The Exercise: Exhale and raise your straightened leg to the height of your bent knee, or get as close as you can. Exhale on the way up (you'll notice a good ab contraction, too) and inhale down. Imagine your heel being pulled to lengthen your leg throughout the exercise.

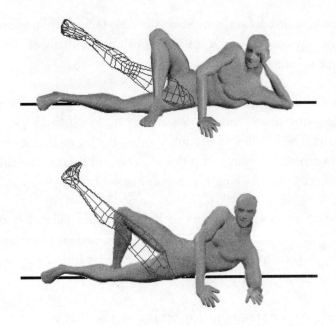

6–13 Inner Thighs (a) Top leg back (b) Top leg forward

Top Leg Forward

Preparation: Assume the same position as above, but instead of resting your weight on your forearm, come down a bit so that you're supported by your elbow, with your hand just under your ear. Cross your bent leg over in front of your straight leg, and your weight will roll from resting on your bun back up onto your side again.

The Exercise: Exhale as you raise your straight leg up. It won't go very far, but you'll still be able to feel the work going on up high in your inner thigh.

14. Standing Hip Flexors

Technical Purpose: To strengthen hip flexors, the most commonly and profoundly weakened muscle among patients who lean back.

This exercise simulates the muscle as it's used when walking and activates the hip flexors from a standing position. It also works your abs for trunk stabilization.

Gait Application: Just as your toes are about to leave the ground into the swing phase, the hip flexors prepare to lift the leg and bring it forward. The hip flexors lift and shorten the leg so that it clears the ground without dragging. Hip flexors, abs, and balance are the combined forces you're looking for to stabilize your trunk.

Preparation: Find something to hold on to for balance and stand next to it sideways. Set your eyes, chin, chest, and ribs slightly down, and stretch your free arm out to the side and a little in front of you with your elbow slightly bent.

The Exercise: Extend one leg behind you so that your toes are on the ground. Put most of your weight on the ball of your standing foot, but don't lift your heel. Keep your foot flat on the floor and your weight forward. Exhale as you slowly bring your knee up to waist height or higher, making sure that the heel and the knee move

6–14 Standing Hip Flexors

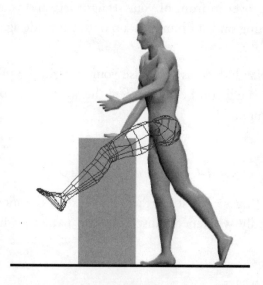

in a straight line up from the floor (don't allow anything to turn in or out). You can also do this with no support (both arms outstretched). That increases the balancing and trunk-stabilization benefits.

15. Half-moons

Technical Purpose: To strengthen the hip rotator muscles in conjunction with work that develops sandwich system strength. This also develops quadriceps (knee) strength.

Gait Application: As you walk, you need to twist while on one foot. This twisting requires knee support and propulsion from your hips in addition to sandwich system strength. They all work together in this exercise.

Preparation: Lay on your back, knees up, feet firmly on the floor a little wider than hip width, with your arms at your sides and your shoulders down away from your ears. If your head is excessively forward or your neck is uncomfortable, you can put a small pillow under your head. Extend one leg straight out. For Outer Half-moons, turn your extended foot so that your inner ankle points to the floor, or is as close to that position as you can get. Later you'll flip your foot the other way so your inner ankle faces up for Inner Half-moons.

The Exercise: This exercise is called Half-moons because you draw the curved part of a half-moon with your heel as you raise your leg straight up. Inhale, then exhale as you lift your leg and twist your heel so you draw an arc, like a crescent moon. When your thighs are parallel (your knees at the same elevation and your leg out straight), you should have completed the crescent. The goal here is to start with your inner ankle down and end up with your inner ankle up, or as close as you can come.

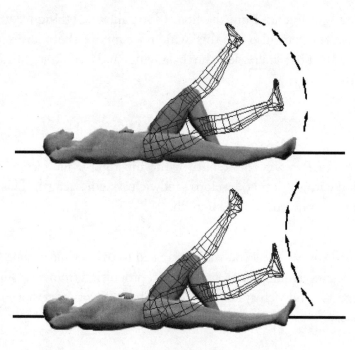

6–15 Half-moons

To do Inner Half-moons, start with your inner ankle facing up toward the ceiling, along with your inner knee, and twist your foot the other way as you raise your leg straight up. Inhale down, exhale up.

16. Hip Extension, Three Ways: Over Pillows, Tray to Ceiling, Hands and Knees

Technical Purpose: To strengthen your gluteus maximus muscle.

Gait Application: People who lean back tend to have little or no muscle tone in their buns, which is where your gluteus maximus lives. This muscle should play a significant role during the pushoff phase as well as at the point at which your weight goes onto your foot at mid-stance. If you're not using your gluteus maximus, you're depending on your hip joints to hold you up.

Over Pillows

Preparation: Lie on your belly with one or two pillows under you the long way. Put your hands under your forehead and have your feet at hip width.

The Exercise: Exhale, flex your foot, and raise your straightened leg toward the ceiling just a little with a short movement. Keep your hip

6–16 Hip Extensions, three ways: (a) Over Pillows (b) Tray to Ceiling (c) Hands and Knees

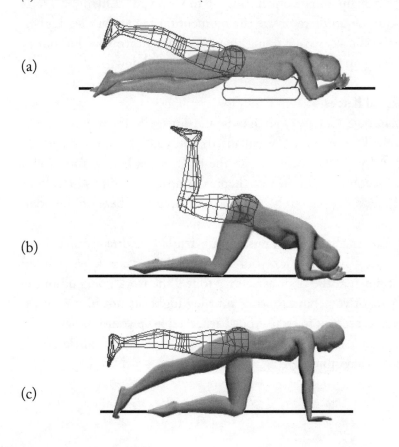

(a)

(b)

(c)

on that side down on the pillow and raise your leg just an inch or so past body height. Inhale down, exhale up.

Tray to Ceiling

Preparation: From a kneeling position, bend over and put your elbows on the ground and rest on your forearms. Your elbows and forearms act as a brace for this one. Put your head down into your open hands (make a little pocket for head support).

The Exercise: Imagine that you're lifting a large tray of cheap, stale hors d'oeuvres to the ceiling with your foot (that way, if you spill a few, you won't be overly concerned). Exhale as you lift one foot toward the ceiling. Inhale and bring your knee back down toward the floor. Exhale up, inhale down. Be sure to keep your belly tight. Don't whip your leg up there or use the momentum to get your leg higher. You can strain your back doing that. Also, don't turn your hip out to get your leg up higher. Just move straight up and down.

Hands and Knees

Preparation: Get on your hands and knees. Keep your back flat (not arched, rounded up, or collapsed) and your chin tucked slightly down, and your eyes centered on the floor beneath you. You should have perfect 90 degree angles where your arms and thighs meet your body. Extend one leg out behind you with your toes bent on the floor.

The Exercise: Exhale and raise your extended leg directly up behind you to body height. Flex your foot and keep your knee pointed straight down at the floor as you try to feel the work going on in the lower part of your bun. Raising your leg higher is not better, and it may even cause you to strain your back. And keep your hips level. Do not shift your hips to the side as you extend your leg. Inhale down, exhale up. Stay sturdy.

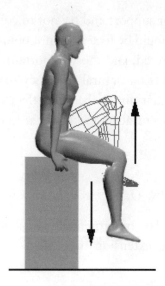

6–17 Sitting Hip Flexors

17. Sitting Hip Flexors

Technical Purpose: To strengthen hip flexors, usually the weakest muscle among patients who lean back. This exercise is done seated so that you can elicit pure hip flexion unassisted by your external rotators. (If you're having trouble sitting due to pain in that position, use Standing Hip Flexors first.)

Gait Application: When your toes are just about to leave the ground, your hip flexors lift your leg and shorten it for forward movement and ground clearance. The focus of this exercise is on lifting the leg forward and straight through as opposed to up and around, which some people do as a substitute for bending at their weakened hips.

Preparation: Sit on something high like a washer, dryer, kitchen counter, or bathroom sink, so your legs can dangle from the knees down. Your knees and feet should be even and at hip width.

The Exercise: Exhale and raise your leg, keeping your knee bent at a 90 degree angle. Be sure to hold your back straight. Use your hands as much as necessary for support and try not to collapse or slouch to lift your leg. Your foot should be flexed up, not pointed down at the floor. Keep your body centered, and most important, keep your foot lined up under your knee. It's a natural tendency to twist your knee outward as it lifts, and that diminishes the effect of the exercise. It can take tremendous concentration to keep that line. This is the place to be vigilant.

18. Opposite Arm and Leg

Technical Purpose: To strengthen the back side of your shoulders, back, and hips using extension movements for all of the extensor muscles.

Gait Application: At the start of each pushoff, a diagonal line of extension occurs that runs from your shoulder, diagonally across your back, and over to your opposite hip. This exercise works to strengthen that diagonal pattern while it builds parts of your upper back and shoulders to undo the adverse effects of slouching or a rounded upper back.

Preparation: Lie over one or two pillows lengthwise. This exercise can be done without pillows, but it's a little harder and can cause a little more strain to your lower back. Put both arms out in front of you, spread to the side at about 45 degrees. Put your legs out the same way. Put one of your feet so the top is on the floor. Put your other foot down so it's resting on your toes.

The Exercise: Exhale and raise your leg (the one resting on your

6–18 Opposite Arm and Leg

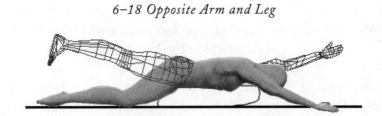

bent toes) and your opposite arm to a level of about one foot off the ground, or as far as is comfortable. Repeat and switch. Your thumb should lead the way to the ceiling.

19. Hands and Knees Balance (Brourman's Balancing Technique)

Technical Purpose: I developed this exercise for a tennis pro who was plagued with shoulder injuries. His weak link (his shoulder) required work that combined balance and trunk strength while he executed rigorous moves on the court. I designed it as a strengthening tool for developing your sandwich system while you move around.

Gait Application: That split second of balance that occurs with each step (referred to in Gait Corrections 2.2, and 4.4) can only be accomplished with back and abdominal (trunk) strength. *Balance and trunk strength are the two main ingredients for a structurally sound gait.* This exercise works on both at the same time, and it also fortifies your legs, arms, and neck. This exercise also works the most important stabilizing muscles as it teaches proper movement patterns.

Preparation: Get on your hands and knees. Keep your back flat (not arched, rounded up, or collapsed) and your chin tucked slightly down, and your eyes centered on the floor beneath you. Your hands and knees should make a perfect little rectangle where they meet the floor. Your feet should be straight out behind you (not turned in toward each other), and you should have perfect 90 degree angles where your arms and thighs meet your body, which is still flat, right?

6–19 Hands and Knees Balance (Brourman's Balancing Technique)

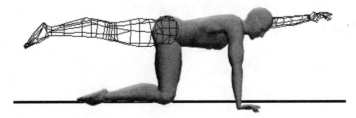

The Exercise: Inhale as you hold still. Then begin to exhale and slowly raise two opposing extremities (for example, your right arm and left leg) straight up to body height. (Higher is *not* better, and try to keep your shoulders and your hips flat, as if there were a ruler on each that you're trying to keep level.) Stay up there and inhale. Hold your belly tight to keep your back flat. Then start your exhale and slowly lower your arm and leg to their original positions. Exhale up, inhale at the top, then exhale down and inhale at the bottom.

The raising and lowering motion should be done softly, with controlled landings. You should return to that perfect rectangle you started with. Stop and inhale, then exhale again as you repeat the raises using the opposite limbs. Like the Cross Crawl, this exercise seems to work better when you don't count repetitions but rather do it for a period of time, like the length of your favorite song or to a timer set for four minutes. That lets you focus on the components of your balancing act instead of counting.

Note: The first time you attempt this, it's okay to practice raising just one arm or one leg to get the proper feel and positioning. Go on to the whole exercise when you're done experimenting. Also, you're going to move your arms and legs around, so maintaining your balance will be tricky. Here's a helpful hint. Since you want your body to stay centered, flat, and motionless as you use your arms and legs, you need to know how to move without shifting from side to side, which will be your natural tendency. To compensate for that inclination, push your standing knee(s) or hand(s) slightly toward each other and down into the ground. They won't actually move, but that pressure will help you keep your balance. Pushing your right hand down and toward your left knee, for example (while your left hand and right knee are in the air), causes you to use your trunk strength to achieve the balance you need without contorting. Careful: no rounding of your back to accomplish the pushing.

20. Standing Balance

Technical Purpose: To teach, reinforce, and strengthen your sandwich system and your capacity to maintain balance on one foot with your weight lifted up and over in the forward position.

Gait Application: This exercise simulates the "split second of balance" you look for in each step (referred to in Gait Corrections 2.2 and 4.4), except you're standing still instead of walking. It is an exaggerated version of what's required as you hold your balance for that split second when your other foot is busy swinging through the air. Your new muscle strength, especially your sandwich system, must be strong enough to hold you up so you can stop depending on those overused joints for support.

Preparation: Stand with your arms stretched out in front of you as if they were wrapped around a giant beach ball. Your chest, ribs, and chin should be relaxed and pointed down slightly, not lifted up high. Pull your head back and put your chin slightly down so you could see the crown of your head in a mirror.

6–20 Standing Balance

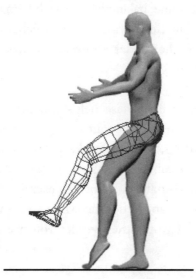

The Exercise: Put one foot out in front of you, with your toes pointing down touching the floor and your heel up. Most of your weight should be on the ball of your back foot, and that knee should be soft. Inhale and then slowly exhale as you raise the front foot, knee slightly out and bent, to about the height of your stationary knee, or as close as you can get. Be careful not to let your shoulders ride up as you lift your leg.

Remember, your weight should be balanced almost entirely on the ball of your standing foot (very little weight on your heel). Inhale at the top and then exhale as you lower your leg to the floor and slide your foot back to standing posture at approximately hip joint width (widened stance). Don't fret if you have difficulty finding your balance. The fidgeting and squirming you do is the very stuff that teaches your body balance. Fight for your balance for as long as you can. Then once you find it, exhale and lower your leg without crashing it to the floor (control the landing).

21. Belly Press

Technical Purpose: To strengthen the abdominal and spinal muscles deep inside the center of your body. This exercise also incorporates your upper and lower abs, and is the basis for trendy terms like "neutral spine" and "spinal stabilization," which I call your sandwich system. Most ab and spine balancing (or stabilizing) exercises incorporate these inner muscles. Grasping the mechanics of this exercise will prepare you for the harder ab exercises that will have an even greater impact on your gait.

Gait Application: This exercise helps you develop the abdominal strength that's required to keep your ribs down when walking, bending, twisting, or lifting. That helps keep your upper body forward when you walk. This exercise works at the core of your body, and it's quite odd in the sense that as part of this exercise you have to flatten your spine. You don't want to do that while you're walking, but when lying on your back it works the muscles you need to get those ribs pointed down.

Preparation: Lie on your back, knees up, feet firmly on the floor a little wider than hip width, with your arms at your sides and your head and shoulders down. If your head is excessively forward or your neck is uncomfortable, you can put a small pillow under your head. In fact, you can use a pillow for any of the floor ab exercises, especially if your chin tends to jut out when you're on your back. After a while you'll want to wean yourself away from the use of pillows.

The Exercise: Inhale, and then slowly exhale as you lower your ribs toward your navel. It should almost feel like you're narrowing your rib cage as you move it down. Make sure that you do this exercise without putting any pressure on your feet and without tightening your buns. Just use your ab and back muscles. Next, inhale and relax your back again. To relax, let your back arch a bit if you want. Inhale, and then slowly exhale as you start the process of lowering your ribs again. Repeat this ten to twenty times.

When I tell my patients to squeeze their backs down into the floor, sometimes they can't figure out what I mean. So I put a towel under the small of their backs and just below their shoulders and tell them to pretend it's their favorite T-shirt. Then I tell them that as they squeeze down, I'm going to pull their favorite T-shirt out from under them, and if I can pull it out, I get to keep it. People really like their favorite T-shirts, so I generally lose (sometimes they think they've won a towel).

Note: Pelvic Tilts, a commonly misunderstood and misapplied exercise referred to earlier in this book, is very similar in its prepara-

6–21 Belly Press

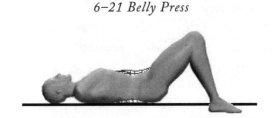

tion but extremely different in its execution. Many of my patients have had to "unlearn" Pelvic Tilts, primarily because it asks that you use your buns and/or feet to assist with the exercise. If you do this during belly presses, you defeat the entire purpose of the exercise. Do not tighten your buns or put any pressure on your feet while doing this exercise. Also, do not suck your belly in. It does not strengthen your abdominal muscles at all.

22. Cross Crawl

If You Have Low Back or Sciatic Pain: The Cross Crawl exercise is especially good for preventing, and even eradicating, low back and sciatic pain. If you currently suffer from sciatic pain, the strengthening process associated with the Cross Crawl exercise (and most ab exercises) ironically requires positions that may exacerbate your situation at first. If you find this to be the case, do Press-Ups, Side Reaches, and Standing Back Bends (along with the rest of your gait correction routine, of course) until you're strong enough to do the Cross Crawl without pain.

Technical Purpose: To strengthen your abdominal and spinal muscles, and to stabilize your trunk in order to create a strong sandwich system.

Gait Application: Develops trunk strength to make staying "up and over" less taxing. Once you grasp the "up and over" concept, you'll find that implementing it full-time requires sandwich system stamina.

Conditioning is necessary, especially if those particular muscles have grown weak from disuse. It's important that you combine the gait corrections and the exercises to accomplish the long-term benefits of genuine structural stability.

Preparation: Lie on the floor with your arms at your sides, knees up, and feet flat on the floor. Your feet should be slightly wider than hip width. To check this, roll your head to both sides to see if you can see your feet. If you can't, widen your feet until you can see them.

Note: If you walk with a narrow base of support, you also may tend to exercise with your feet too close together. A good way to retrain for a wider base of support while walking is to do the floor strengthening work wider, too.

The Exercise: This exercise has two parts that you should practice separately before you attempt them together. Both parts are done on the floor, knees up, feet apart and flat, as described above.

Arm Switches: Put one of your arms straight up overhead, hands slightly cupped with fingers and palms pointing up. (If your shoulder bothers you, put a pillow above, not under, your head to limit the downward descent of your arm and relieve shoulder stretch.) Inhale, and with one arm still overhead and your other arm down at your side, start your exhale and squeeze your lower back down, pressing it into the floor. As you continue to exhale, switch arm positions. When you've finished exhaling, relax your back and inhale. Exhale again as you switch arm positions.

Knee Switches: Start with your arms relaxed at your sides and pull one of your knees up toward your armpit as far as you can comfortably go. Inhale with your knee still held up toward your armpit, and start to exhale slowly as you squeeze your lower back down, pressing

6–22 Cross Crawl

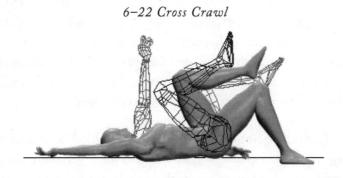

it into the floor. As you continue to exhale, slowly switch your knees. When you've finished exhaling, relax your back and inhale. Exhale again as you switch leg positions.

Arm and Knee Switches Together: After you feel at home with each of these individual exercises, you can combine them so that you are doing one leg and the opposing arm at the same time. Don't allow frustration to arise. All my patients feel like they have flailing, out-of-control limbs when they first try this. Think to yourself, "Opposites up," as you make the arm/leg switch. Inhale, leaving your arms and legs at rest, start your exhale, switch your arm and leg positions, and finish as you complete your exhale. It's better if you don't count repetitions. Instead, work for a specified amount of time, like five minutes. Some patients do this exercise for thirty minutes and more because of its meditative action. If it seems too easy for a five-minute workout, you can add small weights to your feet and hands (start with one pound and move up from there). You can also increase the intensity of the exercise by stretching your down leg flat to the ground each time (it's harder to sustain the back squeeze down, which translates to a better return on your exercise investment).

23. Alternating Knees

Technical Purpose: To further strengthen your sandwich system, specifically the lower part, which consists of your hip flexors and lower abs. This exercise may help you feel the difference between your upper and lower abs, especially when done in context with the belly press exercise. If you do these exercises correctly, it's possible to feel fatigue at two clearly different abdominal areas. Also, this exercise may seem confusingly similar to the knee switches part of the Cross Crawl. The difference is that this one focuses more on lower abs, while the Cross Crawl focuses on the upper and lower abs combined.

Gait Application: Some exercises have the added benefit of incorporating movement patterns that emulate those required for a balanced gait. In addition to strengthening beneficial muscle groups,

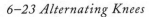

6–23 Alternating Knees

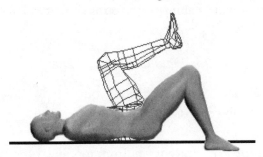

they familiarize you with structurally sound walking patterns. Learning the correct patterns is part of the program. One of those patterns occurs when your hip flexors and lower abs lift your leg in preparation of moving it forward. This exercise strengthens muscles and promotes the proper gait pattern associated with lifting and holding your leg during the swing phase.

Preparation: Lie on your back, knees up, feet firmly on the floor at a little wider than hip width, with your arms at your sides and your head and shoulders down.

The Exercise: Inhale as you bring one knee toward your armpit on the same side. Don't shift your body to facilitate bringing your knee up. Keep both hips down and don't press your other foot into the floor to leverage your knee higher. You should use only the strength of your hip flexor as you bring your knee up as far as you comfortably can without contorting. If it's not easy, don't worry. It gets easier with time. *Don't force anything.* Then exhale and squeeze your back down as you slowly lower your leg to the starting position.

Note: If you're used to walking with a narrow base (your feet too close together) you may tend to lower your leg to a similarly narrow position rather than to the width of your hip joints. Place some object between your feet, like a box of tissues, to give yourself some feedback as to where your feet are landing. The more you strengthen your hips with your feet in the proper widened position, the easier it will be to incorporate that wide stability into your gait pattern.

24. Double Knees to Toes

Technical Purpose: To strengthen your sandwich system, with emphasis on the lower abs.

Gait Application: To prevent you from toppling over, the muscles at the front and back of your trunk co-contract and squeeze you together like a sandwich. The front part of your sandwich system, which is made up primarily of your lower abs, is largely responsible for the "over" part of the up and over gait correction.

Preparation: Lie on your back, knees up, feet firmly on the floor at a little wider than hip width, with your arms at your sides and your head and shoulders down.

The Exercise: Inhale as you bring your knees up toward your chest, making very sure to keep your legs parallel and apart. Exhale as you squeeze your back down and lower your legs with your big toes pointing down just about to the starting position, but instead of coming to a complete halt, just touch your toes, inhale, and bring your knees up again. You should try to touch your toes to the floor as close to your buns as is comfortably possible. As you get stronger, you can extend them out a little farther, which increases the abdominal excursion and thus the strengthening benefit. But beware! If you send those toes out so far that you can no longer squeeze your back down to the floor, you will defeat the purpose of this exercise, and you might strain your back.

Note: To make this exercise a little more piquant, you can bring your head up into the Upper Ab Crunch position for a few reps per set. You can make it even harder by adding weight to your feet or by wearing shoes. If you have excessive hip turnout, you'll tend to bring your legs up and separate your knees too far. That's because your

6–24 Double Knees to Toes

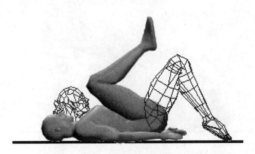

body defaults to familiar patterns. Don't let old patterns dominate. You're attempting to build strength with less turnout, because turnout leads to leaning back. Make sure your ankles are as far apart as your knees.

25. Table Exercise

Technical Purpose: This is done essentially for the same purpose as the Double Knees to Toes exercise, which bolsters your sandwich system. One difference is that this exercise tinkers with your upper abs as well as your lower abs (the Double Knees to Toes exercise is more for the lower abs). They're both good exercises for strengthening the abs without bending your body over or forward. But the Table Exercise is a little safer for your spine, and it more closely emulates positions you'll encounter in everyday life.

Gait Application: Strengthens the sandwich system and thus all things related to your glorious new Primary Movement Pattern.

Preparation: Lie on your back with your legs and knees up at a 90 degree angle, as if you were resting your feet on a table. Put your arms at your sides with your shoulders down and flex your feet so they're also at 90 degrees.

The Exercise: Inhale as you slide your legs in the direction of your body, making sure that the bottoms of your feet face the wall. Move

6–25 Table Exercise

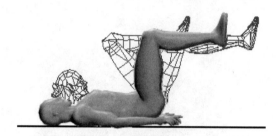

your heels as if gliding along the top of the table, making sure your feet remain perpendicular to the floor (toes pointing to the ceiling). Exhale and squeeze your back down as you slide your feet back away from your body to their original starting point, legs at 90 degrees. Inhale as your feet move toward you, exhale them away from you.

For this exercise, you must keep your back squeezed down to the floor as you exhale (that's when you extend your legs away from you). As a result, you may find that you can extend your legs out only one or two inches past 90 degrees. As you repeat this exercise and build strength and flexibility, you will be able to slide your legs farther and hold them out longer. On the other hand, if you find this exercise too easy, try bringing your upper body into the Upper Ab Crunch position for a few repetitions per set (as shown in illustration 6-28), and/or add weights to your feet (or wear heavy shoes).

26. Low Ab Knee Switchers

Technical Purpose: To strengthen your lower abdominal muscles, along with your hip flexors and quadriceps.

Gait Application: The lower abs, hip flexors, and quadriceps are the muscles that pull your body weight up and over your foot during the stance phase. This exercise strengthens your body so it stays forward. Notice your Sandwich system muscles at work. This helps prevent slouching.

6–26 Low Ab Knee Switchers

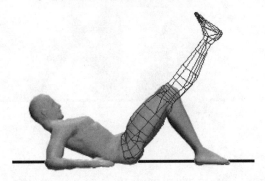

Preparation: Sit on the floor with your knees bent and your feet flat. Lean back so your hands are on the floor just behind your hips, fingers forward, with your elbows slightly bent. Or you can lean all the way back onto your forearms. In either case, keep your back fairly straight. Pick the position that's most comfortable for you (it's easier on your forearms than up on your hands).

The Exercise: Keeping your thighs parallel, exhale as you bring one foot up so your leg is extended straight out. Feel your abs work to keep your back flat as you simultaneously switch your legs. Inhale still, and exhale to switch.

27. Oblique Crunches

Technical Purpose: To strengthen your oblique abdominal muscles.

Gait Application: The strength required to twist your torso and balance your body over the front of your feet as you propel yourself forward depends a great deal on your oblique abdominal muscles. Those are the muscles that pull you to each side, generating that all-important twisting motion from the middle of your body. One set of obliques initiates the twist, and another set halts the twist (otherwise you'd keep on twisting until your skin and bones stopped the twisting motion, and most likely you'd just fall over).

6–27 Oblique Crunches

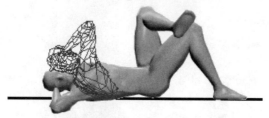

Preparation: Lie on your back with one knee up (foot flat on the floor a little wider than your hip bone), and cross your other leg over so your outer ankle rests on your opposite knee. Put your hand behind your head on the side with your knee up, elbow out, and your other arm out to the side at 90 degrees.

The Exercise: While keeping your eyes on your bent elbow, exhale and bring that shoulder (the one attached to your bent arm) toward your opposite thigh. Your shoulder blades should come all the way up off the floor. Repeat this flip-flopped so you reverse everything for the other side. Do three to five sets of five or ten per side. I like to do combinations of ab exercises, like ten left and ten right Oblique Crunches, then do a few sets of Upper Ab Crunches, and then come back for some more Oblique Crunches.

28. Upper Ab Crunches

Technical Purpose: To strengthen the upper abdominal muscles. When your *upper* abs are weaker than your lower abs, you tend to have a rounded upper back and a concave spine. When your *lower* abs are weaker than your upper abs, your upper body tends to be more stable, but you may tend to favor one side out of habit, thus leading to hip, back, and neck vulnerabilities.

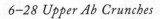

6–28 Upper Ab Crunches

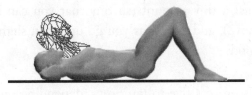

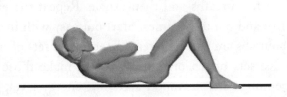

Gait Application: The upper abs play a vital role in keeping you up and over, which is one of the primary gait corrections. The upper abs are situated right at your all-important pivotal point of trunk rotation. That rotational motion (the twist) is also where the power of your sandwich system comes in. Those muscles hold your torso in place at the axis of your body. Strengthening your abs is a primary ingredient of a healthy gait.

Preparation: Lie on your back, knees up, feet firmly planted on the ground a bit wider than your hips. Clasp your hands behind your head with your elbows open and your pinky fingers at the base of your skull (the top of your neck). Alternatively, you can put one hand behind your head at the base of your neck (elbow pointed up), and your other arm can just rest across your belly. This alternative requires greater shoulder flexibility, but the advantage is that it tends to prevent your neck from trying to do the work that your belly needs to do. You can switch sides all you like in the course of your repetitions.

The Exercise: Exhale as you raise your upper body, using the muscles around your solar plexus. Get up as high as you can without bending or curving the small of your back. Make sure your hands stay behind your head (or that your forearm does). Then inhale and go back down just a tiny amount (so tiny that you can barely feel the downward move), and exhale as you go up again slightly. Stay there for a few seconds.

Repeat this process five to ten times, depending on your strength and stamina, and then inhale and go back down to the starting position. Take a few breaths and then exhale. Repeat the entire process between five and ten more times. Start out easy with five sets of five, or less if your abs are weak. Increase later to five sets of six, and eventually to five sets of ten or more. You can make those sets easy or hard, depending on your mood and your energy level, but five sets should be plenty, especially if you are also doing the other ab exercises described in this section.

Note: Unlike your neck muscles, your abdominal muscles are more stalwart and should be exercised rigorously, but not to the point of straining yourself. You can work your stomach muscles until you feel some burning or shakiness in there. This isn't harmful.

29. Sitting Lats

Technical Purpose: To strengthen your latissimus dorsi (or "lats," the muscles at the back of the shoulders).

Gait Application: "Keep your shoulders down" is certainly one of the most common expressions used at my clinic. But many people are unaware that they carry their shoulders high (or forward) in an effort to balance themselves. Your lats come into play on the rear shoulder and arm swing, and if they're not strong and active, either your shoulder looks slouched forward or you get the "held up by a coat hanger" effect. Both lead to structural vulnerabilities.

Preparation: If you have healthy knees, get on the floor and sit on your feet. If your knees give you problems, sit on the edge of a chair.

6–29 Sitting Lats

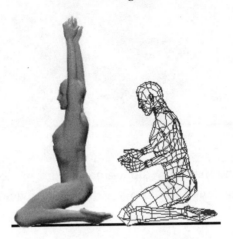

Lean forward a bit with your chin down on your chest, hold your back flat, and extend your arms toward the ceiling.

The Exercise: Exhale and lean your flattened back forward a little bringing your scapula and pecs down. Pull your elbows down and back, bending your arms as you lean slightly forward. Inhale as you bring your body and arms back up again. In this exercise, you need to add or create some internal muscle resistance. I imagine that I'm in water and pushing against a current to simulate that resistance.

30. Modified Push-ups

Technical Purpose: To strengthen your pectoral muscles in combination with your back and ab muscles.

Gait Application: This exercise helps keep your back strong and your belly from hanging out as you use the sandwich system for a structurally sound gait.

Preparation: Get on your knees with your feet crossed at the ankles. Have your arms straight, your belly tight, your back flat, chin in, eyes on the floor. If you are sure you can keep your back flat—with no buns

6–30 Modified Push-ups

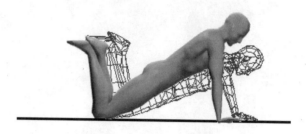

sticking up and no belly slouching—you can do regular push-ups on your toes instead of on your knees. Or you can do some of each.

The Exercise: Exhale as you lower yourself by bending at your elbows. Your elbow bend may be as little as 15 degrees in the beginning, or you may be able to lower your nose all the way to the floor. You have to feel this one out and do what you can without straining. When done on a regular basis, your strength and endurance will build up quickly and noticeably. It's good if you feel some level of fatigue after completing this exercise. In fact, a burning sensation in your muscles is a sign that you're building them up. But don't overstrain. You can tell if you're correctly exerting yourself the next day. If you are not sore, do more.

31. Scapular Push-ups

Technical Purpose: To strengthen your pecs, rhomboids, and serratus anterior (the muscle that holds down your shoulder blades).

Gait Application: People who lean back sometimes develop the unfortunate habit of trying to hold themselves up by their shoulders. As noted earlier, this can make them appear to be held up by a coat hanger. Their shoulder stabilizers (the muscles that hold their shoulder blades down) have simply grown weak. When I get a patient like this I put my hands on the shoulder blades and tell the patient to relax and let the

6–31 Scapular Push-ups

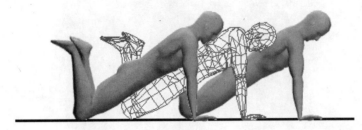

shoulder blades spread across the back. They seem surprised to learn that such movement potential exists in their shoulder blades. Soon they discover that walking around as if they're expecting a sharp slap on the back is not a good thing.

Preparation: Get on your knees, with your feet crossed at the ankles. Have your arms straight, your belly tight, your back flat, chin in, eyes on the floor.

The Exercise: Keep your elbows straight and lower your upper body using your shoulder muscles. Keep your belly tight and your back as flat as possible as you drop down and come back up.

32. Back Shoulder Rolls

Technical Purpose: To strengthen your rhomboids and lats, and to stretch the front (pecs) and top (levator and upper traps) muscles of your shoulders.

Gait Application: Having the strength to pull your shoulders down and back is especially important during back arm swing, and to some extent throughout your shoulder rotation (your arms augment twist and forward motion). Also, when you lean back, your head and shoulders tend to come forward for balance, something you want to avoid. This exercise helps you develop square shoulders that stay down and back automatically.

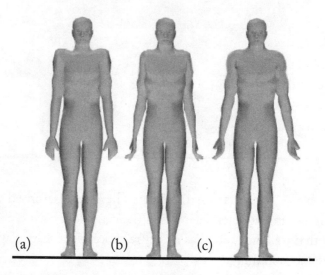

(a)   (b)   (c)

6–32 Back Shoulder Rolls (a) Up (b) Back (c) Return (notice hand positions)

Preparation: Stand in front of a mirror, either facing it or sideways (you'll actually want to do this exercise both ways so you can see how it affects you from both angles).

The Exercise: Allow your arms to hang at your sides and pull your shoulders up, then roll them back, and then squeeze them down and back. Return to the starting position, with your arms hanging at your sides, and repeat.

33. Neck Flexors

Technical Purpose: People who carry their heads out in front of their bodies lose strength in their neck flexor muscles. When your head sits up on your shoulders correctly, it's held in place above your torso by the front neck muscles (neck flexors) and the back neck muscles (neck extensors). Keep in mind that your head is more like a bowling ball than, say, a balloon, so imagine the work required in trying to keep it from plopping over when it sticks out in front. Gravity does everything in its inexhaustible power to pull your head, and everything else, down. And what's preventing that? Instead of sharing the burden with all your neck muscles, the neck extensors at the back of the neck get stuck doing all the work.

As the muscles at the back of your neck perform a double shift, neck pain often results, as does tension in the shoulder blades. This also explains most double chins. When the neck flexors go to sleep, which they tend to do because they've been told they're free to go on vacation, they grow weak. That area of your neck may tend to be fleshy and sag. This exercise rescues your neck extensors, not to mention your entire gait.

Gait Application: The ability of your head to stay up is really quite amazing. Ever see a person on the street with a body that appears to be sideways, but a head that looks straight up and down? Your inner ear, and your eyes, are extremely willful and act like an internal gyroscope to keep you perpendicular. Because of that, when you begin to correct your structural balance by bringing your weight to the balls of your feet, your head automatically (but slowly) tends to go back into the position where it belongs, directly above the shoulders.

Because your neck extensors have been dormant for so long, they may get sore quickly if you abruptly bring them back out of retirement without preparation (exercise). In order for your neck flexors to resume 50 percent of the workload of holding up your head, they need to get in shape, but take it slowly.

Preparation: Lie on your back, knees bent, feet firmly planted on the floor a little wider than your hips. Make sure that your shoulders are down as explained in Gait Correction 6.4, not up around your ears.

6–33 Neck Flexors

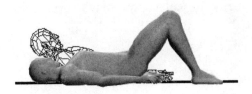

The Exercise: Inhale and lie still. As you exhale, tuck your chin down slightly (leave enough room between your chin and your chest for a small apple). Then raise your head, bringing your chin closer to your chest. Stay up in that position and inhale. Then exhale and lower your head back down to the starting position. It's imperative that you *tuck* your chin down slightly during this exercise in order to make sure you're strengthening the correct muscles (don't stick your chin out).

Note: Neck exercises tend to be more strenuous than others, so don't overdo them and risk ending up with a sore neck. Do just a few of these to start out with and increase in tiny increments, like one or two a week. You can start with a pillow under your head to decrease the workload if your neck is weak or you encounter discomfort. You can even start with two pillows, which will further reduce the distance your head moves, thus making the exercise less strenuous and less of a threat.

34. Neck Extensions

Technical Purpose: To strengthen the muscles at the back of your neck, which are responsible for half the work of holding your head up and back.

Gait Application: A forward head can be a manifestation of leaning back, or the cause of it. Either way, the muscles that hold your head up and back have to be strong enough to do their job comfortably or you'll be tempted to revert back to a forward head. Also, weak neck extensors can force you to use your upper shoulder muscles to hold up your head, which gives some people that turtle look, an unbecoming configuration. The turtle look is the result of muscular weakness, not genetic misfortune. Sometimes you'll notice the turtle look on really muscular guys, maybe even weight lifters. That just means they overworked the back side and underworked the front side of their necks.

6–34 Neck Extensions

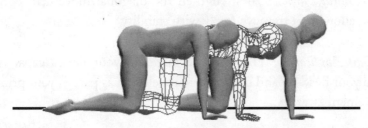

Note: In the last exercise (Neck Extensors) you learned that it was important to exercise the muscles at the front of the neck because they're probably weak. Among people who lean back, the muscles at the front of the neck are generally weaker because the muscles at the back of the neck have been doing all the work. Now we're telling you that it's important to exercise the muscles at the back of the neck, too. So you might wonder why that's necessary if they're already over-worked. The answer is that your neck flexors (the muscles at the back of your neck) may be strong with your head in a forward position, but not very strong with your head back where it belongs. It's important to exercise your neck flexors with your head up and back so those muscles develop strength for that particular position.

Preparation: Get on your hands and knees. Keep your back flat (not arched, rounded up, or collapsed) and your chin tucked slightly down, with your eyes centered on the floor beneath you. Your hands and knees should make a perfect little rectangle where they meet the floor. Your feet should be straight out behind you (not turned in toward each other), and you should have perfect 90-degree angles where your arms and thighs meet your body.

The Exercise: Inhale and drop your head toward the floor without moving anything else, keeping your face parallel to the floor. Exhale as you pull your head back up toward the ceiling, still keeping your face parallel to the floor. Start with three sets of five.

35. Side-Lying Neck Rotations

Technical Purpose: To strengthen the diagonal movement of your neck, allowing it to move freely with stability.

Gait Application: This exercise increases your neck's capacity to hold your head up and back, where it belongs, as part of your primary movement strategy.

Preparation: Lie on either side with your legs mirroring each other (or with your top leg forward and resting on the floor). Rest your ear on your arm and put your other arm in front of you on the floor so your hand can brace your body.

The Exercise: Bring your head forward and touch your forehead to the floor in front of you (or get close). Then bring your head back and touch the back of your head to the floor behind you. Repeat, but remember that all neck exercises need to be treated with more cau-

6–35 Side-Lying Neck Rotations

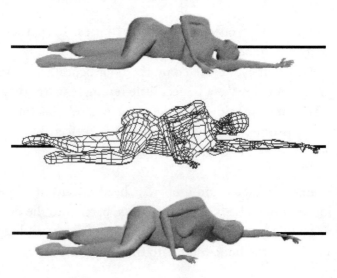

tion, so go easy and start with just a couple of repetitions and then move up. To make this exercise easier, use your free arm (the one your head is not resting on) to help with the lifting power needed. Just push your free hand into the floor and that pressure helps your neck muscles lift your head more easily. You can make it even easier by placing a pillow behind your arm, so that when your head goes back, it has less distance to travel.

36. Neck Diagonals

Technical Purpose: To strengthen neck muscles, specifically the stern-ocleidomastoid muscle, which helps hold your head up and back. The technical purpose of this exercise is basically the same as for the Neck Flexors exercise. This exercise, however, is particularly applicable if your neck is in pain or if your neck needs special attention. It helps strengthen your neck faster and more thoroughly than most other neck exercises.

Gait Application: As with the Neck Flexors exercise, Neck Diagonals help strengthen the neck muscles you use to hold your head up correctly, directly over your shoulders.

Preparation: Lie on your back, knees bent, feet firmly planted on the floor a little wider than your hips. Make sure that your shoulders are down as explained in Gait Correction 6.4, not up around your ears. Turn your head to one side as far as comfortably possible. For comfort and protection, you can start with a pillow under your head

6–36 Neck Diagonals

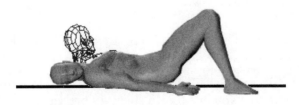

and neck. With pillows this exercise requires less work, so lose the pillows as soon as you can.

The Exercise: Do this exercise the same way as the Neck Flexors. With your head to the side, bring your chin slightly down (as with the Neck Flexors exercise, leaving enough room between your chin and chest for a small apple). Exhale as you turn and lift your head up so you're toward the opposite side of your chest. Stay up there as you inhale, then exhale down to the same side on which you started. (If the breathing part messes you up, you can exhale up and inhale down.) When you're at the top looking over the other side of your chest, your chin should be pointing to the breast of the opposite side from which you started. Just do a few on each side to start off.

37. Belly Press with Sideways Breathing

Technical Purpose: This exercise teaches you the proper way to breathe in order to keep your weight forward while you walk.

Gait Application: Walking with your weight in front of you requires that your ribs be down inside your abdomen and that when you breathe, your ribs move outward, not upward. Improper breathing mechanics are often the culprit behind gait deviations. When you breathe down into your belly or straight up into your chest, that tends to throw your weight back. That, of course, leads to leaning back when you walk.

Preparation: Lie on your back, knees up, feet firmly on the floor a little wider than hip width, with your arms at your sides and your head and shoulders down.

The Exercise: This is a four-count exercise: (1) inhale and relax; (2) exhale, squeeze your back down to the floor as in the Belly Press exercise; (3) this is the hard part: inhale, but keep your back squeezed down (note that you just took a sideways breath!); and (4) exhale and squeeze down harder. As you squeeze down harder, you will be strengthening the sandwich system again, but this time in a functional way, because those same breathing mechanics teach you how to breathe so you stay forward on your feet while you walk.

38. The Groucho Marx

Technical Purpose: Strengthens your quads and hamstrings to facilitate soft-knee walking. Strengthens your ankles, specifically the anterior tibialis and peroneals.

Gait Application: Improves balance in the forward position, which is where you want your weight: forward, not leaning back. This exercise forces you forward on your feet so you can't lean back.

Preparation: Find an area to walk around in without many obstacles.

The Exercise: This is called the Groucho Marx because he used to walk around crouched down just for a hoot. I doubt that he knew he was strengthening his quads and hamstrings at the same time. Anyway, keeping your feet wide, and remembering to twist your body as you walk, crouch down slightly by bending your knees more than usual. Walk around like that for three to five minutes, staying down low while incorporating your gait corrections. You'll find that the lower you go the more strength and balance is required and the more you tend to stay forward. The more balance you force upon yourself during this exercise, the more you'll benefit.

39. Tip Toes

Technical Purpose: To strengthen your calves, specifically the gastrox/soleus muscles, in conjunction with your quadriceps. This exercise also strengthens the arches of your foot.

Gait Application: People who lean back tend to lose their pushoff. This exercise simulates how your muscles work at the beginning of pushoff, when the hip flexors (the psoas muscles) are stretched almost as they'd be if you were up on your tiptoes. It also strengthens your calves, also used during pushoff.

Preparation: Stand up on your tiptoes as high as you can get, and try to prevent your heels from going in toward each other, as they would if you turned your knees out too far (headlight knees pointing too far out).

The Exercise: Walk around on your tiptoes. But make sure that your upper body twists and that you have the proper arm swing, just as a healthy gait should have. Don't flap your arms around or forget all the other things you've learned. Stay forward and twist, just like walking. This exercise is best done for an increment of time—like the length of a TV commercial or while you're getting dressed in the morning. It's even okay to do standing still, but it's better to walk. This exercise improves the shape, strength, and tone of your calves. If your calves are too skinny or flabby, this is a great way to build them.

40. Heel Walk

Technical Purpose: To strengthen your shin area (anterior tibialis muscles).

Gait Application: People who lean back tend to rush their swing phase and barely clear their feet off the ground as they walk. At the start of the swing phase, the foot's ability to pull up properly requires the participation of muscles located in your shins. In fact, this exercise is especially good for healing shin splints (which indicate that you lean back when you walk). *Although it's unlikely that you lean back when you run, your Primary Movement Pattern, and subsequent structural vulnerabilities, are mostly determined by how you walk.*

Preparation: Get up on your heels. Go for it.

The Exercise: Start by walking around for two minutes or so and work up to five minutes. This can be a pretty mindless exercise, so do it while you're in the kitchen or clearing dishes or something. Really pull your toes up when you're on your heels. Those muscles you feel are the ones that help you lift your foot.

41. Slo-Mo Walking

Technical Purpose: This exercise is multipurpose. You can do it to improve virtually any aspect of your gait that needs work (balance, knee strength, to find the axis of your twist, to get to know the proper forward lean, to find a comfortable eye line-of-focus).

Gait Application: Any and all.

Preparation: Get your body into the correct position by lifting up and over, unlock your knees, bring your weight to the front of your feet, and envision taking long, wide steps. You're ready.

The Exercise: This is just slow-motion walking, folks. The sequence breaks into four parts: (1) step and extend; (2) lift and lock; (3) twist and face your shoulders toward your forward leg; and (4) step down wide.

6–41 Slo-Mo Walking

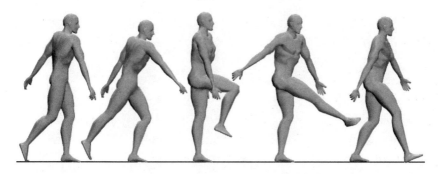

In more detail: First, take a step and bend your standing knee a little more than normal. Leave your back leg extended behind you a little longer than usual, too. Let your back heel stick to the floor a bit
like there's gum on it. Raise your back foot off the floor slowly and
extend your arms (one forward and one backward, of course) a little
more than normal. Hold this position for a couple of seconds. Second, bring your back leg forward just to the center, where your knee is
bent in front of your foot underneath. Lock in your balance by focusing your eyes twenty feet ahead of you and pressing your palms down,
fingers outstretched to the sides. Hold this for a couple of seconds.
Third, staying balanced, slowly twist your trunk and switch your arms
so that your shoulders are facing the leg that's about to move forward.
Fourth, step forward with your feet at hip socket width. You have to
really bend that standing knee in order to step down wide without
losing your balance. Keep Slo-Mo Walking for two minutes.

⊰ 7 ⊱

STRETCHING EXERCISES

EXERCISES THAT CORRESPOND TO YOUR GAIT CORRECTIONS

Stretching exercises offer your body all kinds of benefits.
 I have started off many lectures and seminars saying, "Flexibility is the spice of physical life and what keeps these bodies young. If you get stiff, you get old fast."

Stretching is a softening, loosening manipulation that actually allows muscles to increase in length. Strengthening muscles, on the other hand, usually makes them harder or tighter. For simplicity's sake, think of stretching as softening and strengthening as toughening. While strengthening exercises build muscles for a balanced gait, stretching exercises make them pliable in a way that's equally conducive to a balanced gait.

STRETCHING BY-LAWS

As with any exercise program, it's impossible to come up with one routine that fits everyone. But some general principles apply, most of which were provided in Chapter 6, Strengthening Exercises under "Strengthening By-laws (page 116)." Please familiarize yourself with that section.

With stretching, you need to be able to "feel" the difference between underdoing it and overdoing it. When you don't stretch enough, it feels rather empty and void of muscle feedback, and when you stretch too much, it feels painful and forced. Once again, the appropriate level of exertion requires knowing that "sweet threshold of pain" that only you can recognize.

Frequency and Repetitions

The best way to accomplish lasting results is to stretch frequently, at least three times a day, doing three repetitions per stretch. That's my "3-by-3 Rule." Some patients focus on one particular stretch per week, fitting in others when they can. If you can stretch only once during the day, you'll still get positive results. But keep track of what your muscles are doing the other twenty-three and a half hours, and recognize that to maximize results you need to spread stretching work out during the day much like your gait corrections.

Like the strengthening exercises, stretching exercises can be done anytime. Strengthening and stretching work well together. Some people prefer to stretch before exercising to help them warm up. Some like stretching after they exercise to maximize stretching benefits, since warmed-up muscles stretch more easily. Some stretch before and after exercising. As long as you stretch, consider it valuable whenever you do it.

Never "bounce" to accomplish more repetitions when stretching. In fact, never bounce, period. When you stretch out a muscle briefly and let it snap back, you don't get much value out of stretching, and it can even bounce back to a shorter length. Long, slow reps produce the most beneficial results. In general, I recommend holding a stretch for a count of ten—not speed counting. Also note that a tiny change in angle can give you better stretching results. Recheck your movement constantly, noticing every degree of every repetition.

When a stretch is described for just one leg or arm, we're assuming you know that you need to do the other leg or arm the same way.

Breathing

Let the oxygen in with nice deep breaths. Inhale for relaxing moves, exhale for the stretch. Muscles and tendons love oxygen. And the body is simply softer and more malleable when you breathe with long, slow, relaxed breaths.

I love the "whisper breath." It's an ancient yoga technique that lengthens your breath a lot. In the whisper breath, you limit the airway at the back of your throat by pulling your tongue back and you make this hissing noise that sounds like Darth Vader with his helmet off, or that thing in the *Exorcist*. Breathing like that is good for strengthening exercises, too, but it helps stretching tremendously.

I've had patients use a metronome to measure their breathing, since each exhale should take about a third longer than each inhale. Proper breathing is a process that improves with practice and patience.

Fear and Pain

Some people are frightened at the slightest sense of discomfort; they methodically understretch, sometimes for years. They attempt the positions but never effect a change in muscle length. I frequently hear things like "Stretching doesn't work on me." Baloney.

Learning to feel and read your own body can be difficult, especially if you've been taught to trust advertisements, parents, and doctors more than your own experiences. Start small and stretch into some discomfort a little at a time, and see how you feel the next day. If you are a little sore, that's far enough. Keep that up until you're not sore. That's when you can safely go a little bit further.

You should not experience much more than mild soreness from stretching. If you need aspirin from stretching, you pushed too hard. It's easier to hurt yourself stretching than it is strengthening, but not if you pay attention to your body. Remember, however, that strengthening exercises push your endurance threshold more than your physical dimensions, which are clearly more finite. As for stretching too often (as opposed to too hard or too far), it's rare to find people who are overstretched. If they are, they're usually overstretched due to a structural weakness.

Diet

For increased flexibility, muscles should have a high-mineral diet and lots of fluids. Drink lots of water to provide the necessary muscle elasticity you need. Eat foods that grow in the ground for natural minerals. You can certainly take this further by incorporating dietary supplements into your routine. I take them by the handful.

Okay, go stretch!

List of Stretching Exercises

STRETCHING EXERCISES

1. Calf Stretch on Wall

Technical Purpose: To stretch the gastrox and the soleus muscles.

Gait Application: Just before pushoff, your lower leg muscles need to be flexible. That allows your heel to stay down long enough to create that sublime second of balance that leads to strengthening in all the right places.

Preparation: Stand about one and a half feet from a wall. Reach out, placing both hands on the wall, step forward with one foot and backward with the other. Keep your feet pointed straight ahead.

Gastrox Stretch: Bend your forward knee so that you're really leaning into the wall. Make sure both feet remain pointed straight forward, perpendicular to the wall. Depronate your feet as much as possible (don't roll your feet in). Move your back foot as far back as

7–1. Calf Stretch on Wall (a). Soleus (b). Gastrox (c). Start Position

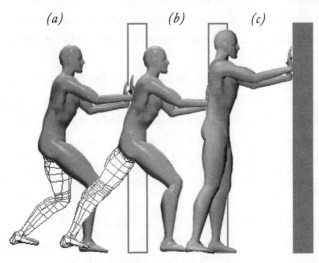

(a)   (b)   (c)

you can without lifting your heel and without rolling your feet in or out. Alternate with the Soleus Stretch, below.

Soleus Stretch: Bring your back foot forward, maybe halfway in, and move your front foot a little closer to the wall. Keep your hands on the wall (the push will feel a little lighter) and bend both knees. That will make you feel as if you're sitting down with your buns sticking out. Now lean back on your back foot. I like to switch back and forth between these two poses a few times before switching sides.

2. Clock Stretch

Technical Purpose: To stretch your entire spine, trunk, hips, and shoulders in rotational and diagonal patterns.

Gait Application: Flexibility is essential to the trunk rotation and diagonal patterns that make up your new gait. The other main ingredient is muscle strength, but here we're just working on increasing your flexibility.

Preparation: Lie on your side with your head resting on your bottom arm. Bend both legs and put your top leg a little forward of your other leg. Stretch your top arm straight out in front of you on the floor.

The Stretch: Imagine that you're lying on a big clock and your top arm is the big hand. Stretch your top arm out to three o'clock, but stretch it even farther so you can feel the stretch come out of your trunk more than out of your shoulder joint. From there, point at the four, then to every remaining number on the clock. The bigger the circle you make, the better. Work it like a dance. Let it flow, and allow your body to roll back to get to the nine, and when you're getting toward the six, lift your head, using your bottom arm for all the support you need. I even get up on my elbow at that point and reach like crazy. Do that three times in each direction, on each side, for a total of twelve reps.

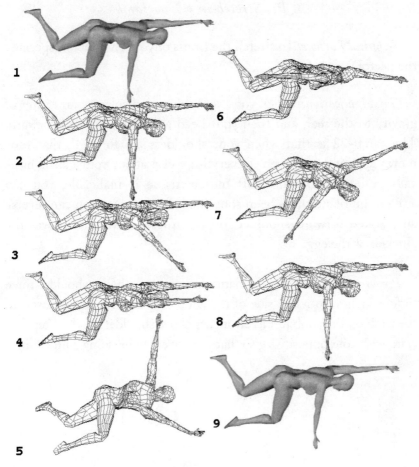

7–2 Clock Stretch (aerial view)

Note: If you have a sore shoulder, you can cut some corners by making your arm movements less intense. Also, if you've had back or neck pain, do this very gingerly at first. Start slowly and feel at each new reach whether you need to lessen the amount of stretch to make it safe for yourself.

3. Pec Stretch in a Doorjamb

Technical Purpose: To stretch the fronts of your shoulders, especially the pectoral muscles.

Gait Application: When you lean back, you displace your center of gravity to the rear, and then your head and shoulders roll forward. The catch-22 is that when your shoulders are forward, that promotes leaning back, even if everything else about your gait is basically realigned. Because soft muscle tissue is malleable, you can stretch the tissue that's been shortened. By doing so you can reverse an adapted forward shoulder roll regardless of whether it was the chicken or the egg.

Preparation: Stand in a doorjamb facing out with one shoulder three to four inches from one side of the jamb. Put the arm that's closest to the jamb on the jamb just a few inches above shoulder height. Step forward with your opposite leg so that you appear to be doing a little lunge.

7–3 Pec Stretch in a Doorjamb

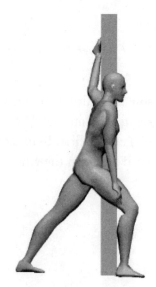

The Stretch: Slowly inch your front foot forward to increase the stretch at your shoulder. For those of you with shoulder pain, be careful because this turns out to be a fairly aggressive shoulder stretch. Move your foot slowly over the course of this exercise, and use caution. Feel this one out.

4. Seated Back and Neck Stretch with Shoulder Rolls

This is definitely one of the safer stretches, so relax and allow yourself a little more movement than you're used to.

Technical Purpose: To gently stretch the whole spine using forward, backward, side-to-side, and diagonal movements.

Gait Application: The ability of the spine to move with ease in all of these directions is not only a primary ingredient to a well-balanced PMP but the best way to decrease vulnerability for all types of spinal injuries. As you learned in Chapter 3, when part of your spine is rigid or stiff, even a small mishap can have a negative impact that could have been avoided if your spine had greater flexibility.

Preparation: Sit at the front edge of a chair, feet flat on the floor supporting you and at about hip width. Put your hands on your lap.

Note: A common mistake during neck stretches is to drop *just* your head (forward, back, or to the side). That's not good because all of the stretching gets focused at one spinal level. That can overstretch some areas and totally neglect others. Neck stretches should run throughout the spine simultaneously at multiple levels, creating nice curves, not 90 degree angles.

Forward and Backward Stretch Gently bend your spine so that it's rounded. Then slide your weight into your thighs and arch your back. As you arch, continue to look straight ahead (you'll get to extend your

7–4 Seated Back and Neck Stretch with Shoulder Rolls (a) Diagonal Stretch (b) Seated Shoulder Rolls (c) Forward and Backward Stretch (d) Side-to-Side Stretch

(a)

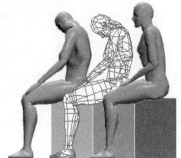

(b)

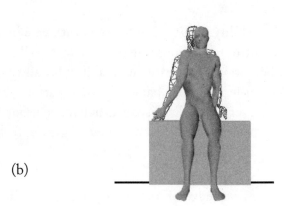

(c)

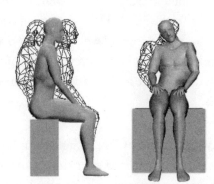

(d)

neck in Standing Back Bends, but don't do it here). Round and then arch your back several times.

Note: This is a lot like a slouch except that you aren't collapsing into it from weakness, you're purposely contracting into a rounded spine from your tailbone to your neck. This takes belly work—as opposed to slouching, which takes no work.

Side-to-Side Stretch Slide all your weight over onto one bun as you drop the ear on your other side to the shoulder on the same side. Shift from side to side several times, alternating buns and ears.

The Diagonal Stretch Shift your back out to one side and drop your head over to the opposite side with your nose pointing down at your armpit. Come up and reverse everything to the opposite side. Repeat several times. This can be awkward because you're probably not used to moving this way, but this exercise feels great when done correctly.

Seated Shoulder Rolls This is just a natural progression of the Diagonal Stretches. That is, you'll want to follow the Diagonal Stretch with the Seated Shoulder Rolls once you get the hang of them. Roll one shoulder up, back, and then down while the other one moves down, forward, and then up. Keep this opposing rotation going for ten turns or so, and then reverse directions.

5. Wall Stretch Routine

There are three parts to the Wall Stretch Routine, all accomplished from the same start position. As you become familiar with how each one works, you can combine or resequence them. If you're healing from a strained back or neck, some stretching routines can compound your problems, but not this routine. It's safe. I do it when I'm reading the newspaper. It just seems like a good idea to be sort of

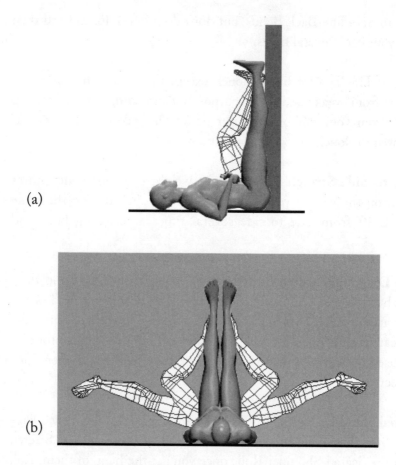

(a)

(b)

7–5 Wall Stretch Routine (a) Hamstring Stretch (b) Frog or Hip Stretch

upside down for a few minutes every day. It lets gravity work in reverse.

Preparation: Find a wall that you can sit down in front of and put your feet up on. The idea is to have your back and buns down on the floor, with your legs up on the wall, your body bent as close to 90 degrees as possible. Getting into position can be an exercise all by itself. Sit close to the wall, a little sideways to it, and then roll down on an elbow and gently throw your legs up onto the wall, heels centered (not turned in or out). Make sure your shoes don't mark the wall—or better yet, just remove them. And make sure there's enough wall space for you to spread your legs out into a big V shape.

Hamstring Stretch

Technical Purpose: To stretch the hamstrings in a position that leaves the lower back out of the stretch, safeguarding it via the support of the floor.

Gait Application: At heel strike, the length of your hamstrings permits (or limits) the fluidity and extent of your stride.

The Stretch: Slide your heels up to the point that you feel a gentle stretch on the back of your thighs or the back of your knees (some people's hamstrings are tighter at the top, near their buns, and some are tighter at the bottom, near their knees). Don't worry if either (or both) of your knees are bent, or if you can't get your buns down on the floor with your feet up on the wall. That just means your hamstrings and low back are *really* tight—and this is the best and safest way to begin changing that. Go slowly and let gravity do the work. You don't have to push hard. That's the whole point of the wall and being sort of upside down. The longer you stay there, the more gravity works for you. Flex your feet for even more limbering benefits. Read the Sunday paper with your feet up on the wall.

Frog or Hip Stretch

Technical Purpose: To warm up your hips, especially your hip internal rotators (gluteus medius and minimus) on the way up, and your external rotators (gluteus maximus) on the way down.

Gait Application: Your hamstrings stretch more easily after the hip joints are warmed up. Plus, striding with long, balanced steps cannot be accomplished with tight hamstrings.

The Stretch: Slide your heels up and down on the wall several times (knees open) holding that stretched position for ten seconds or as long as a minute.

Inner Thigh Stretch

Technical Purpose: To stretch the adductor longus, magnus, and gracilis muscles.

Gait Application: The width of your steps is powered by the inner thigh, so it needs to be strong and limber to provide the wide base necessary for proper balance. Without it, you'll tend to lean back and take a seat in your hips. Relying on the genius of your joints to hold you up, instead of muscle strength, is a threat to structural health.

The Stretch: Slide your heels out to the sides, making sure that your knees continue to face straight back. Don't turn them in or out as you slide, even if you can only go out a little way. Stay out there so you feel your inner thighs stretch for ten to fifteen seconds at first, and alternate with the other wall stretches. Allow a gentle adaptation to take place for those body parts of yours that may never have been stretched before. You may want to begin doing one side at a time. Then go for the big "V"! Once warmed up, I enjoy moving back and forth between the hamstring stretch and the big "V."

6. Supine Stretch Routine

The Supine Stretch Routine relaxes the body, and it's a quick way to stretch most of your major muscle groups. This stretching routine consists of several segments, each of which flows well from one to the next with little or no break. You should do three reps on each side, which will take only a couple of minutes once you catch on. The results can be marvelous if you really get into this one with your heart and soul. When I get frazzled, this keeps my whole body from seizing up. I do this routine at night before bed, and it's been quite handy during the laborious hours spent giving birth to this book.

7-6 Supine Stretch Routine

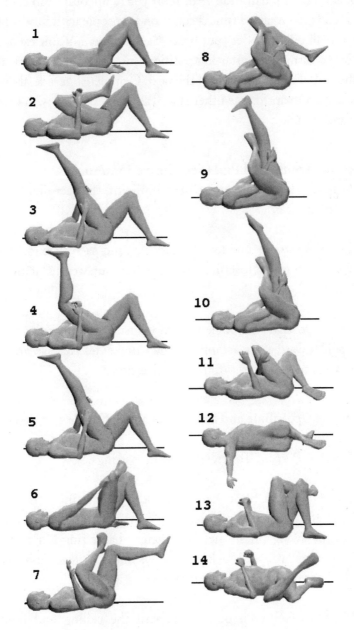

Preparation: Lie on your back with your knees bent, feet flat on the floor and separated about the width of your hips. Put your arms at your sides (See illustration 7–6, 1). If you're uncomfortable, or if your chin tends to be raised (this is common for people with forward heads), put a small pillow under your head. Each segment of this exercise ends *without* returning to a starting position. Just string each segment along so the end of one is the start of the next. Complete one side, then switch legs and do them for the other side. Take long breaths with each position and stretch.

Knee-to-Armpit and Pull (See illustration 7–6, 2)

Technical Purpose: To stretch the hip joint, the sacroiliac joint, and the lower back.

Gait Application: The lower back, hip, and sacroiliac joint have to be flexible in order to efficiently transfer your weight at the end of each pushoff.

The Stretch: Lift one knee toward yourself, grab it with two hands, and pull toward your armpit on the same side. Release and repeat, same knee to same armpit, three to five times

Extend It Up, Inhale and Soften the Knee, Exhale and Stretch (See illustration 7–6, 3, 4, 5)

Technical Purpose: To stretch your hamstrings.

Gait Application: Short hamstrings lead to back injury because they pull you aft, begging you to lean back. At pushoff, your lead leg (the one in the swing phase) needs sufficient hamstring length to stride out, otherwise you will tuck your pelvis under instead, and that leads to a loss of your natural lumbar curve.

The Stretch: Stretch one leg toward the ceiling and hook your hands behind your knee. Make sure you stretch gently, without putting stress on your back. Inhale and soften your knee, exhale and stretch your leg and knee. You can push your other foot into the floor for better leverage and use your hands to help straighten your leg (be careful not to overstretch).

Bring It Down, Cross It Over, Press It Open (See illustration 7–6, 6)

Technical Purpose: To stretch the piriformis muscle.

Gait Application: Folks with huge foot turnout often find that their piriformis muscle is way too tight. In fact, sciatic pain can be caused by that alone. Stretching it can dismantle the pain. If the relief seems to be just temporary, it's probably because your old pattern is still reinforcing the tightness. Fixing it comes with time, patience, and commitment.

The Stretch: Let go of your knee and bring your leg down until you can cross the ankle over to the other knee. Use the hand on the same side to press your knee open with gentle pressure. Hold this for about five seconds, and press and exhale a couple of times.

Raise Crossed Legs, Grab the Leg Underneath, and Raise It to Stretch Your Ankle (See illustrations 7–6, 7, 8, 9, 10)

Technical Purpose: To further stretch your piriformis, hamstrings, calves, gastrox, ankle, and anterior tibialis muscles.

Gait Application: This stretch is beneficial for the same gait applications described above. Plus, this stretch helps the ankles limber up, which is important at the very end of the stance phase. People with tight calves often have a bounce, or what's called a vaulting gait, because they pop up a little too fast. By itself, it's the least offensive of all the possible gait deviations, but since it's usually associated with short hamstrings, it's worthy of attention.

The Stretch: Press your elbows into the floor to help raise your legs so you can quickly grab the back of your knee (of the underneath leg) with both hands. You can use your elbow to help push your turned-out knee open a little more to further stretch the piriformis muscle. Then raise the underneath leg (the one that's not crossed over) to further stretch your hamstrings. At the same time, inhale and stretch your toes to the ceiling. Exhale and stretch your heel to the ceiling to stretch your calf and ankle. Let go with your hands, bend your knee, and slowly bring the foot you've just stretched to the floor.

Cross Your Top Leg All the Way Over, Drop Legs to Side, and Turn Your Head the Opposite Way (See illustrations 7–6, 11, 12)

Purpose: To stretch your outer hip muscles, especially the tensor fascia lata (TFL), and gently stretch your entire spine with a spiral staircase motion.

Gait Application: By now you know the consequences of an inner heel strike. People with tight TFLs often have an inner heel strike and a wider base on the floor, as this muscle pulls their legs straight out so they look like an upside-down V. The spinal twist in this stretch works the spine from top to bottom, including all its surrounding musculature, to enable the rotation necessary in a balanced gait.

The Stretch: As you cross your top leg all the way over, use your opposite hand to pull it down to the floor. Extend your other arm in the opposite direction and turn your head to look at it, thus creating a complete spinal spiral staircase stretch.

Note: Since you're already on your side, this is a good place to insert the Clock Stretch. The Clock Stretch is a little more rigorous.

Press Your Elbows into the Floor, Unravel Your Body, and Uncross Your Legs (See illustration 7–6, 13, 14)

Use your elbows for leverage as you untwist your body back to your starting position—back down, feet flat on the floor. To safeguard your back, use your elbows to support yourself as you unravel.

7. Sitting Stretch Routine

This is a bit more advanced than the Supine Stretch Routine because it requires lower back and hamstring flexibility just to get into the starting position. If you've been having back pain, and especially leg

7–7 Sitting Stretch Routine

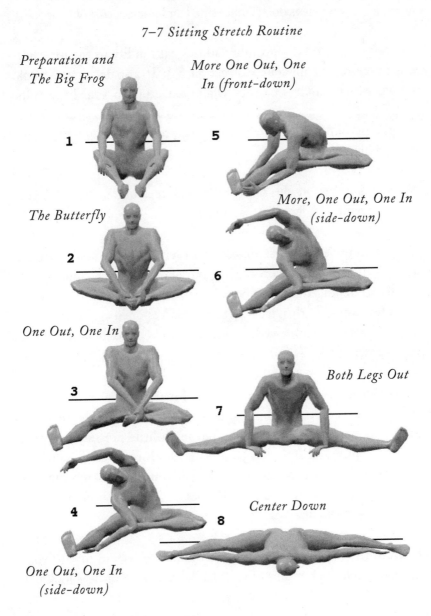

Preparation and The Big Frog

1

The Butterfly

2

One Out, One In

3

4

One Out, One In (side-down)

More One Out, One In (front-down)

5

More, One Out, One In (side-down)

6

Both Legs Out

7

Center Down

8

pain, this routine could irritate surrounding nerves and worsen the pain. Stretch with caution.

Technical Purpose: To help increase your natural lumbar curve by stretching your hips into external rotation and your lower back into extension while in the seated position. (Please note that the external hip rotation going on here is done while seated and not as a part of your gait.)

Gait Application: Hip flexibility adds great fluidity to the hip-slide motion referred to in Gait Correction 5.1. It also facilitates trunk rotation, which requires balance when you're up on your little stilts (legs). When done correctly, walking with muscle-based balance strengthens your body with every step you take. Walking with joint-based balance does not.

Preparation: Sit on the floor with your feet out in front of you about twelve inches, legs bent, and knees out.

Note: If muscle tightness makes this one too hard, don't push it, and don't despair. Start with one leg out and one leg in, and experiment by stretching over your bent knee instead of the straight one. After a few weeks of this, try it with both knees open again. Remember, this is a slow, snail-paced, powerful process of adaptation, so you need to accept progress in tiny steps.

The Big Frog (See illustration 7–7, 1) Inhale and relax, and while keeping your back straight up and down, exhale and open your knees (get them closer to the ground) by putting a little pressure on them with your hands and by using your outer thigh muscles to help pull them down. Hold them down so you feel your inner thigh muscles stretch for a few seconds; repeat five times. I like to roll back and forth to vary my lumbar curve.

The Butterfly (See illustration 7–7, 2) Pull your legs in toward your body and touch the bottoms of your feet together. (Your legs look like butterfly wings, right?) Hold on to your feet and don't worry if your knees face up like the wings of a closed-up butterfly. It may take a while to comfortably open up. If you experience discomfort, redirect your focus from the tightness in your groin and/or inner thighs to the work you feel in your outer thigh when you extend your knees toward the floor. Try to use your outer hip muscles even more. Work into that for a few breaths, exhaling down, inhaling up, and relaxing. Then go to the next position.

One Out, One In (See illustrations 7–7, 3, 4, 5, 6) Put one of your legs out straight and pull your other foot in toward the other knee. Bend over to the side, placing your lower arm on your inner thigh. (This is the side down position.) Reach up and over with your upper arm sideways in the direction of your straight knee. Exhale going down and inhale coming up. Turn your body so you're facing your straight leg. (This is the front down position.) Slide both hands under your leg and very gently pull yourself over as you exhale; inhale again as you come up. Return to the side down position and move back and forth between front down and side down. Now you're ready for the hardest part, but you can start off as small as you like.

Both Legs Out (See illustration 7–7, 7) Open both legs up so they're straight out. Spread them as far apart as you can without hurting. Worry about spreading them farther later on, but make sure you get to that point of "sweet pain" that tells you you're really stretching something. Work in this position by leaning to both sides and rock forward and back. Slide your hands down the sides of your leg on both sides, and finally, if and when you're ready, go to the last position.

Center Down (See illustration 7–7, 8) First of all, *don't* do this if you're having back or leg pain of the structural type. If you aren't, work your way down slowly by using your elbows for support. Wiggle back and forth between your hips to keep the extension and continue with the lowering. Use your belly strength and exhale as you come up. Use your hands as necessary.

8. Press-ups

Technical Purpose: Another stroke of genius that emerged from Dr. Robin McKenzie was an exercise that proved to be a godsend for me as a therapist. As a spine patient myself, it spared both me and my patients a lot of pain, not to mention that it offered a great body-balancing tool for improving your gait. This exercise helps with leg pain, neck pain, and lower back pain. It works best when used at the onset of pain. When pain has been present for a while, it requires more repetitions to unravel the discomfort and may take a much longer time or even some outside intervention.

Gait Application: Besides reducing pain, this exercise helps you to concentrate on the proper movement patterns. It reduces nerve compression as it stretches the entire spine to the point of extension and flexibility it was intended to have. Like the Standing Back Bends, it helps to restore your natural lumbar curve, which allows your trunk to hoist and twist more easily while walking. When the curve is absent, you tend to lean back and walk without any twist, and that leads to trouble.

7–8 Press-ups

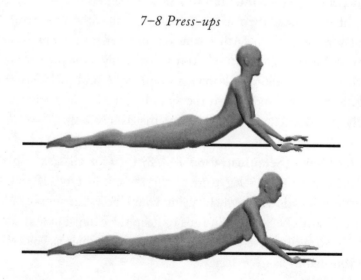

Note: Even though your chest puffs out while doing press-ups, this action is not desirable when walking. This exercise helps increase flexibility, which increases your ability to lift your upper body and twist it properly as you walk.

Preparation: Lie on your belly. Place your hands under your shoulders as if you're preparing to do push-ups. Where you put your hands is less important than your comfort, so move your hands around according to what works for you as you lift your body. I'm happiest with my hands a bit wider than my shoulders at about ear height..

Note: If you do this exercise with preexisting leg pain, then just lie still for a few minutes and allow your body to settle into the extension. It may seem that this position is causing the pain. If you can relax, the pain should subside as you rest or during the repetitions.

The Exercise: With your spine relaxed and soft, raise your upper body by pushing up with your arm muscles while allowing your trunk to collapse. This is one of the few times you actually want your belly to be like jelly. The more back curve you get, the better. This is a passive exercise working on your back, so don't use your back muscles to do any lifting. The lift is generated by your arms. When you start doing this exercise, you may be able to go only a few inches up. That's fine. Some people can straighten out to full arm's length. Eventually you may, too. It will also help you to bring your shoulders down toward your waist, relax your back, and gently lift your chest while keeping your neck long as a giraffe's.

For people in pain, I generally recommend doing at least fifteen to twenty-five repetitions of this exercise five or six times a day. For people in no pain, or just a little, you can get away with less. Incidentally, doing this exercise first thing in the morning (even before you get out of bed) is a good idea if you wake up in pain. It's also a good idea to do these before bed and after any activity that might cause leg pain, like sitting in a certain position for too long. Try a few and mix them up with Standing Back Bends.

Note: Once again, it's important to remember that if you have pain, you should let it (and common sense) be your ultimate guide. If your pain persists, you may need additional help. If possible, obtain help from someone whose education includes training in Dr. McKenzie's techniques.

9. Standing Back Bends

Technical Purpose: To increase the flexibility of your spine and to create traction or distraction to separate the vertebrae, giving more space to disks and nerve roots to decrease nerve compression and leg pain.

Gait Application: As I've mentioned before, many people are taught to eliminate their lumbar curve by tucking their buns under. It's very important to have that natural lumbar curve, especially while walking. This exercise hoists your upper body up off the hips to bring out that natural curve. For those of you who are used to tucking your buns under, this is a great way to begin to lift and extend the spine, thereby untucking your buns. When walking with your upper body lifted correctly up and over, the pelvis (and therefore the buttocks) naturally falls into place.

Preparation: Stand with your feet slightly wider apart than your hips. Place your hands behind you and clasp them at the small of your back. Your feet should point straight ahead (don't turn them out for this exercise, and you *do* want to lock your knees).

The Exercise: Slide your hips way forward and then lift your chest up toward the ceiling. Then drop your head back so it's relaxed.

Note: This is one of Dr. McKenzie's original exercises, which his patients do as often as a few hundred reps per day. I don't often prescribe that many, but it can be a significant pain reducer, and if you are experiencing sciatic pain, I recommend you do these spaced out

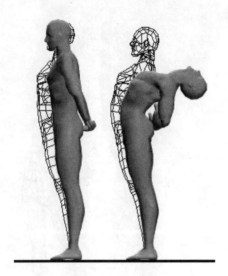

7–9 Standing Back Bends

throughout the course of your day (for example, ten of them, seven times a day). Lifting your chest up while doing this exercise decreases neck problems that can occur when doing this exercise. However, as with all exercises (especially this one), be careful if you already have neck pain. *Begin slowly, and if it bothers you, decrease the duration or intensity, or discontinue the exercise altogether.*

10. Hip Slider Reaches

Technical Purpose: To decrease any reflex shifts you've developed, to reduce quadratus muscle spasms (probably the single most common cause of back pain), and/or to bring uneven hips into symmetry.

Gait Application: A balanced gait stems from a stable trunk. A stable trunk has symmetry from front to back, from side to side, and through both diagonals (shoulders to opposite hips). Back pain commonly starts with a spasm in a muscle called the quadratus, which sets off several chain reactions that can intensify to the point that it's

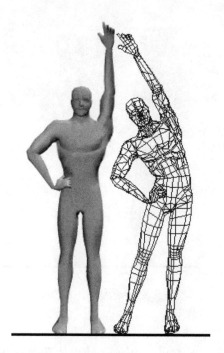

7–10 Hip Slider Reaches

no longer easy to discern what started it all. The most common result is a subtle shift away from the painful side, which leads to a high hip and one leg that takes a narrow step. All of the gait corrections are much easier after you have brought symmetry to your hips and spine, which this exercise helps make happen.

Preparation: Stand with your hand on your high hip (it's detectable in a mirror), feet apart, knees soft, weight in the front of your feet.

The Exercise: Use the hand on your high hip side to gently slide your hips over to the opposite side. As you do that, raise your opposite arm and reach over your head. Bend at the waist, slightly toward the high hip side. Hold for a few seconds and then straighten. This can be painful for the first several reps, but your body should adapt so that the pain diminishes. If it doesn't, stop and get help from someone who is versed in Dr. McKenzie's work.

11. Hip Flexor Stretch

Technical Purpose: To stretch the front of the hip, especially the psoas muscle, which flexes the hip, and the quadriceps muscle, which flexes the hip and extends the knee.

Gait Application: At the end of the stance phase (as you execute pushoff), the front of your hip really has to stretch out in order to twist and transfer weight to the next long step. That all has to happen while you're staying up and over. This exercise limbers up those hip and loin muscles to make that easier.

Preparation: There are three ways to do this: one is easy; one is harder; the last is hardest. If you have had (or currently have) knee problems, do these only the easy way, unless you're very careful with the harder ways (take it slowly to see how it's working for you).

Easy way: Stand next to a railing, table, wall, or something else you can use for support. If you're using your left arm for support, raise your right foot behind you so you can grab it with your right hand. If that's hard, you can put a towel or strap around your foot so that you don't have to bring it up as high.

Harder way: Lie down on your belly (you can be up on your elbows) and raise your foot toward your bun on the same side. Use your hand on that side to grab your foot at the top of the ankle.

Hardest way: Start down on all fours (hands and knees) and bring one foot through to where your hand on that side is. Do this on a soft carpet or an exercise mat to prevent knee pain. Reach back and grab your rear foot at the top of the ankle with your arm on the opposite side.

Note: It's important that you only attempt this version of the exercise (the hardest way) if you have the flexibility to work with your weight forward on your thigh and not up on your kneecap.

The Exercise: Easy way: While keeping your bent knee pointing down and slightly behind you, gently pull your foot toward your buns. As you pull your foot, do so in such a way that the sole of your

(a)

(b)

(c)

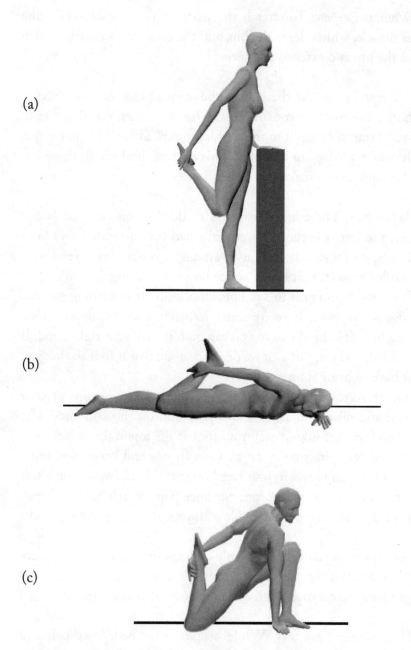

7–11 Hip Flexor Stretch (a)easy way (b) harder way (c) hardest way

foot faces your bun. Keep your standing leg slightly bent at the knee, weight forward, and keep your body straight up and down.

Harder ways: Whether you're on your belly (harder way) or on your hand and knees (hardest way), you should be holding your foot with one of your hands in preparation for the exercise. Pull the sole of your foot closer to your buns to get the stretching effect at the front of your hip.

8

BODY LIVING LESSONS

TIPS ON STRUCTURALLY SOUND WAYS TO APPROACH OTHER DAILY ROUTINES

This chapter will give you information on how to incorporate your new walking mechanics into all your day's activities, including tips on how to:

- get out of bed in the morning
- get dressed
- stand in the bathroom to shave, brush your teeth, and wash your hair
- do kitchen chores such as cooking and loading the dishwasher
- do household chores such as cleaning and vacuuming
- lift objects
- get in and out of a car and drive without neck stress
- sit in and rise from a chair
- sit at a computer
- watch TV
- garden
- do baby care

Remember Terry, his three kids, his happy wife, and their wonder-dog, Boone? Life has returned to normal for them. Terry corrected his Primary Movement Pattern, greatly reducing the likelihood that I'll see him in my office for anything other than a friendly visit.

His overall well-being is not just attributable to his new gait, either. After all, his life includes more than walking. Terry stands, sits, sleeps, eats, shaves, and incessantly picks up Boone's slobbery rawhide chew. Each of these motions can be done with structural salubrity, or they all can be done randomly and without immediate concern or understanding of the long-term ramifications.

Terry used to travel down the road of least resistance, never using much of a sandwich system and always setting himself up for a mishap. Eventually, he had one. It was *the way* he bent over that finally sent him over the edge. I must reiterate that his gait, which contributed more than anything else to his adverse Primary Movement Pattern, was the main culprit behind his structural vulnerability. But Terry made other motions during his daily routine that were just as dismal and potentially damaging. The way he bent over to move Boone, for example, without bending his knees or distributing his weight properly, was all it took to royally tweak his back.

After the Boone escapade, Terry became one of my most dedicated patients. That is, he was curious about the principles of motion I talked about, well beyond just walking. He was particularly curious about the bending over part, since that's what sent him to me in the first place.

I gave Terry a short course in "Body Living Lessons," which is a list of how to do things without hurting yourself. I've been to Terry's house for dinner and watched him cook, clean, bend over, reach, and move in such a way as to confirm my fondest hopes that he has surely grasped virtually every lesson on that list.

I'm going to use Terry's daily routine to exemplify the right way to go about accomplishing the mundane things most people do daily. Like get out of bed. Who doesn't? But how many of you tighten your belly as part of getting up?

MORNING ROUTINES

Terry reports that he tightens his belly as he sits up in bed. In fact, he's in the habit of tightening his belly every time he changes from sitting to standing (or standing to sitting), whether he's getting into a car, sitting down at his desk, or getting out of bed. Excellent.

He doesn't tighten so much that he gets a stomachache. He just stabilizes his trunk and gives his sandwich system a light workout with virtually every move he makes. Terry says that even when he puts his socks on he keeps his belly tight as he practices balancing with most of his weight toward the balls of his feet.

The two bathrooms at Terry's house are always chaotic at 7:20 in the morning. That's mostly because Boone knows that within an hour he's going to be left alone as his playmates rush off to school and work. So Boone tries to crush past anybody who enters the bathroom (or any other room) for fear he'll be left behind. Once Boone has been ushered to the kitchen for his breakfast, Terry showers, shaves, puts in his contacts, brushes his teeth, blow-dries his hair, and twenty minutes later relinquishes the bathroom to his wife and Boone.

While in the bathroom, Terry stands with his knees soft, and he sways from side to side with most of his weight on the balls of his feet rather than collapsing back on his hip joints. When he hurt his back, Terry found that leaning over the sink exaggerated his back pain, so he got a shower mirror that allows him to shave without leaning over the sink. He gave the mirror up when he discovered he could shave by Braille, feeling his face for where to shave. When he puts in his contacts, he goes to his closet mirror so he doesn't have to lean over the sink again. Even though his back has recovered, he recognizes the unnecessary stress that leaning over places on his lower back.

When in the kitchen, Terry is aware of the little moves he makes while standing, reaching, or bending over. He loads the dishwasher, for example, with a new approach. He doesn't bend over at the waist, using his back muscles to hold up his torso. He stands with his entire body in the act, bending his knees, keeping his center of gravity in the middle, with tight abdominal muscles that rescue his lower back.

While we're on the topic of standing and back pain, please note that whether you're standing in line, having a conversation with someone, in an elevator, or upright anywhere, you should sway from side to side with most of your weight on the balls of your feet, keeping your knees soft (not locked). The swaying part is important because when you stand for a long time with both feet flat on the floor, especially if you lock your knees or lean back, you're amassing pressure and placing an awkward load on your weakest parts, generally your neck or lower back. Also, most folks end up over on one side and it's usually the side with the weaker hip! That just aggravates the situation.

HEIGH HO, HEIGH HO

When he gets into his car to go to work, Terry tightens his belly, turns his back to the seat, bends his knees, and lowers his body into the seat without sticking his rear end way out. Once in, he swivels his legs around forward and waves good-bye to Boone and family, waving and wagging at the window.

When he drives, he's not hunched over the steering wheel, either. He keeps his torso straight, using the backrest, and his head isn't sticking out in front of him. His chin is down and his head is back. When he checks for oncoming traffic, he uses his arm to help support his body as he turns his head. If he's looking over his right shoulder, he puts his right arm on the console. If he's looking over his left shoulder, he puts his left elbow on the armrest or the windowsill. That distributes the twist to more levels of his spinal column than the act of simply twisting at the neck. It also reduces *overtwisting*, and that prevents pain.

When he gets to work, Terry brushes the dog hair off his pants and sits down at his desk in the correct way. He tucks his buns under before he sits (that's one of the only times it's okay to tuck them under). Terry puts his chin down and keeps his eyes focused in the

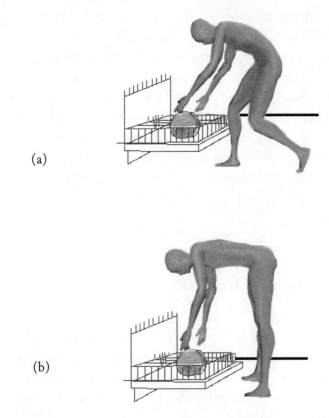

(a)

(b)

8–1 (a) Correct way to load dishwasher (b) Incorrect way to load dish-
washer

direction of his feet. This combination tends to promote abdominal squeeze and the proper weight distribution. He separates his feet so that one foot is farther out in front than the other, which reduces strain on his lower back. He bends at the knees and lowers himself straight down, bending over just slightly as he descends.

Terry used to sit down by bending over and sticking out his rear to meet his swivel chair. He also looked up as he sat down and kept his knees straight. Both of those moves put a lot of strain on his lower back. Oops, isn't that where he had that bad problem?

Terry sits properly, too. His upper body is like a cylinder. He doesn't-sit up high with a big inward curve in his lower back. He doesn't

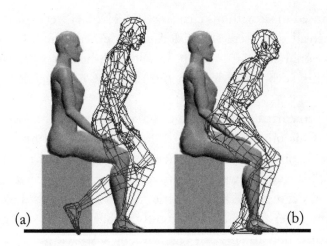

8–2—(a) Correct way to rise from seated position (b) Incorrect way to rise from seated position

slouch or slump with a big outward curve, either. Both of those positions violate the structure of the cylinder. Terry sits lifted with his back slightly curved and his stomach lightly held in.

Terry learned to subconsciously hold his stomach in all the time. At first it took conscious effort while he was learning and strengthening. After a while he just did it naturally. You, too, will develop a strong sandwich system (referred to perpetually throughout this book), and people will tell you how lucky you are to have been born with such nice posture.

WORK HABITS

As an electrical engineer, Terry has his nose relatively close to a computer all day. He sits in one place for hours at a time. As a result, he's learned to shift around in his chair, from side to side, and do mini versions of the back stretch exercises. The ultimate solution, however, is to get up and wander around every so often.

Terry used to sit with his chair too low. His feet weren't flat on the floor. Instead they were all twirled up underneath him. Sometimes his legs would even go to sleep. In addition, he had to reach up to type on his keyboard, which in turn brought his shoulders up too high.

Now Terry has everything adjusted at his desk so he looks down slightly at his monitor (he used to look up at it) and his arms rest comfortably on his desk so his shoulders are down and relaxed. The height of his chair allows his feet to rest flat on the floor with his legs bent at 90 degrees. He keeps a little footstool under his desk to put one or the other foot on intermittently throughout the day, and he's even learned how to cross his legs without any back threat. It's simple: he doesn't slouch anymore. He leans over, resting on his elbow, but he keeps his abs engaged to keep that sandwich system going for a few extra seconds of micro-workout.

There are always project documentation and software disks lying around everywhere in Terry's office. The floor of his office is like a big filing cabinet, but without the cabinet and only one shelf. Terry used to walk around his office crouched over looking for stuff, and that was bad enough on his lower back. But the worst part was how he bent over to pick things up. Somebody once told him that it was a good idea to hold his back straight when he bent over, so he kept his back flat. Ouch. These days, however, he picks things up the right way. He drops his chin, puts one leg out in front of the other a little, and bends at the knees with his buns tucked under his torso. His buns don't stick out as he lowers himself, and he works his knees and his belly instead of his back.

HOME SWEET BOONE

When Terry goes home, he usually takes his briefcase, which is easy to identify from all the rest because Boone chewed part of the leather

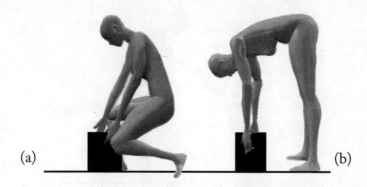

(a)   (b)

8–3 (a) Correct way to lift (b) Incorrect way to lift

handle off. When it's packed with manuals, Terry's briefcase gets heavy, but he has learned to use his legs and his stomach muscles to generate the lift. Terry also knows from experience that lifting his briefcase (or a suitcase when he travels) is best accomplished with his knees bent, the same way he picks up disks from the floor. (I haven't seen Terry pack a suitcase, but I'd be surprised if he stands with his legs straight, bent over at the waist, filling it up with clothes.)

As a general rule, the closer you can get to what you're lifting, the better. Make sure your belly muscles are engaged before you lift or lower, and exhale. Even when you're at the store reaching up high for something, get as close as you can to it. Look down when you put the object in your cart so you don't end up standing there with locked knees, back on your heels, as you lower a five-pound bag of whatever using all your most delicate muscles. Keep your chin down, buns under, and *bend your knees* ("BYK," as we say at the clinic).

AROUND THE HOUSE

When Terry vacuums the house, it really tickles me. He listens to Italian operas, which he plays really loud to overpower the noise of the vacuum cleaner and Boone's howling. After his back problem had

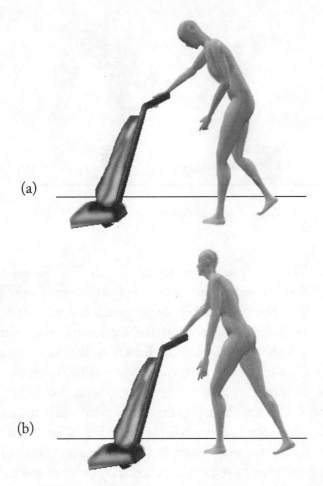

(a)

(b)

8–4 (a) Correct way to vacuum (b) Incorrect way to vacuum

nearly healed, his wife begged me to offer Terry suggestions on how best to vacuum without reinjuring his back. That was easy: use more belly muscles and fewer back muscles. Pulling the vacuum back is simple if your belly is tight and your chin is down, but the pushing part requires you to put one foot out in front of you. Keep both your feet working and keep them pretty close to each other. The trouble comes when you end up on one foot, either pushing or pulling. The main thing to remember is to step forward with a little lunge, use your belly and leg muscles instead of your back, and keep your chin down.

Terry does the household sweeping to rock and roll music. He says it works better than opera. And when he does the dishes, he always keeps his knees soft and his chin down as he loads and unloads. Terry also makes the bed in the morning. (Can you see why I like this guy so much?) When his back was thrown out after the Boone attack, he told me it worked really well to get down on his knees to tuck in the sheets and straighten out the comforter. It helped him keep his belly tight and his back straight. He never had to bend over, so he avoided the back stress that everybody attributes to making the bed in the morning. Now I make my bed kneeling down sometimes, too. Try it.

Besides being a great cook, Terry likes to garden. He grows basil, chives, tomatoes, eggplant, and too many other goodies to mention here. Now he has also mastered the science of structurally sound gardening. The stooping and reaching is not good for you, and it can mess up your neck, back, hips, knees, and whatever else you've got. I can tell by watching him that cushy ground mats and gardening stools are truly great. When I used to weed, I put pillows between my calves and the backs of my thighs and sort of sat and kneeled on them. Either way, the important thing is that you get as close as you can to the plant or weed you're working on. The shorter the distance between you and it, the less leverage you're letting work against your body. When getting up and down, put one foot in front of the other, buns under you, chin down, and drop to, or raise up from, one knee. Use your hands, and keep your belly tight. Also, get up and stretch (do a few Standing Back Bends every fifteen or twenty minutes).

As for watching TV, Terry used to have a big warm cushy chair that he loved to plop down into. But it didn't keep his back straight. Even a couch might need pillows to hold your back straight. It doesn't have to be perpendicular to the floor, just straight. Keep in mind that you don't want your tailbone to slump away from you with a pelvic bend toward your knees. The best way to accomplish that is to have a sturdy backrest. In bed you can lie back on a bunch of pillows as long

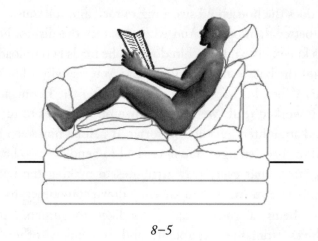

8–5

as there's enough support to prevent a rounded low back or neck (see illustration 8-5).

PREGNANCY AND HANDLING BABIES

This one really yanks my socks off. Terry and his wife have a baby. Guess who changes the little pumpkin's diapers? Yep. And he does it the right way, too. When he carries the baby to the changing table (or wherever), he does *not* carry his baby daughter on his hip, because I've told him (and he can feel) that it's detrimental to his back. Terry puts her on his shoulder (not sitting up there perched, but in his arms with her chest and head on his shoulder).

As far as transporting babies around town, once again, it's not a good idea to use your hip as a shelf. Maybe if you had a baby on each hip it would balance out, but if you don't have twins and a third arm, use a front pack (or a back pack).

Terry takes his baby out of the crib the same way you should lift anything that's out in front of you (groceries from the car trunk, a briefcase from the floor, Boone's spilled kibble). Once again, keep those buns under, keep the chin down, and get as close as you can to the object being lifted, with your feet as close as you can get. The perfect combination for throwing your back out is straight legs, flat back, head up.

Terry even helped his wife avoid the "pregnant waddle" by showing her how to walk without leaning back. It's important more than ever during pregnancy to stay forward on your feet. When you're pregnant, your ligaments are appropriately loosened in preparation for delivery, an act that requires some unusual stretching. But during pregnancy, if you lean back when you walk, your presoftened ligaments are twice as vulnerable, and it's your spine that gets the double whammy. If you stay forward, you'll save your body. Plus, you can strengthen those sandwich system muscles while carrying that extra weight.

SWEET DREAMS

Sleeping is a time to heal. At least it should be. But Terry used to wake up in the morning stiff. His back and shoulders were sore, partially due to his sleeping position. A lot of people scoff at the notion of repositioning their bodies while in the middle of dreamland. They say it can't be done. Oh, ye of little faith!

I told Terry about an interesting way to sleep that I thought might minimize his incessant leg movement at night and reduce his aching in the morning. You lay half on your front and half on your side, with a king-size pillow holding you from collapsing at your midsection (see illustration 8-6, b). So it's only when you actually flip sides that you make a commotion in bed.

It turns out Terry already slept this way—to some extent. His normal style of sleeping was on his side, but with his top leg bent and flopped over so his body faced down. His top shoulder and hip (a)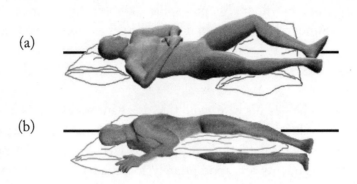

(b)

8–6 (a) Supine sleeping posture (b) Side-lying sleeping posture

never touched the mattress. So as soon as he fell asleep and totally relaxed, his lower back collapsed, which caused his hips, neck, and lower back to fall into an unhealthy position. For Terry, that meant he woke up with a stiff neck and a sore back.

The solution is to wedge a pillow into your lower torso so it doesn't collapse toward the mattress. It's supported by the pillow instead. I also recommend another pillow between the knees. You can adjust your legs, one up, one down, so long as your belly is supported (one big long king-size pillow can do the midsection wedge and the legs all at once, and spooning your partner for the required support can replace the pillows altogether).

When Terry gets out of bed in the morning he doesn't just spring up haphazardly. First he tightens his belly muscles. He uses his arms and shoulders to stabilize his body so he can swivel his legs off the bed and onto the floor (see illustration 8–7).

Some people have actually told me that of all the things I taught them, this sleeping posture was the most valuable tool for reducing their pain. The key is to keep the pillow squashed into your belly so your back doesn't collapse down to the mattress. That's how Terry sleeps now. Combined with all his other structurally correct habits, Terry knows how to successfully walk *and sleep* himself well.

Sweet dreams.

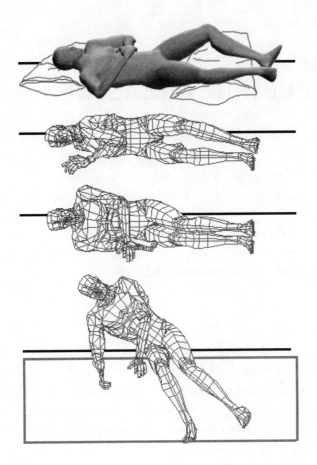

8–7 How to get to and up from side-lying posture correctly

SPECIFIC AREAS OF PAIN

NECK, SHOULDERS/UPPER BACK, LOWER BACK, HIPS, KNEES, ANKLES

This section uses concepts and terminology that will not be totally clear to you unless you've read the rest of this book. If you've just flipped to this chapter, you can still get a feel for what can be achieved, but a complete understanding requires that you read and understand the earlier chapters.

E ach of the stories in this section deals with a person's specific area of pain: neck, upper back and shoulders, lower back, hips, knees, or ankles. The stories are told within the context of each person's gait deviations, which are the result of five variables: daily habits, environment, illness and injuries, exercise history, and genetics. What lies between the source of a gait deviation and a particular area of pain is physical vulnerability in the making. That vulnerability can be traced to elements of the Primary Movement Pattern, the way in which a person walks.

As you read these stories, pick out the elements of each person's Primary Movement Pattern and imagine how and why each one led to their particular area of pain. You'll be able to follow their individual histories and the evolution of their personal profiles in the context of the particular gait corrections and exercises they used to rebalance their bodies and dismantle their pain. Each story concludes with a chart. Each chart summarizes the person's personal profile (Primary Movement Pattern), the gait corrections used, and the exercises the person did, over the course of several months.

Most of these folks ended up (as you will) with stronger, more fluid physical characteristics, not to mention a greater awareness of their bodies and how their problems manifested in the first place. As for *your* pain, there is a chart in Appendix C (page 277) that will help you gauge the intensity of what you're experiencing. Learning to not tense up from pain is a process in itself. If you open up to the process, you can use your pain (as most of the people in this chapter did) as a doorway to a lighter, more balanced form of existence. Pain does not have to be an external force that sets your course of action. Instead, pain can be used as a tool for you to use in setting your own course of action.

When pain arises in the body, it is very common to close around it. But our resistance and fear, our dread of the unpleasant, magnify pain. It is like closing your hand around a burning ember. The tighter you squeeze, the deeper you are seared.

Stephen Levine, *Who Dies?*

Learn how your daily habits, environment, illness and injuries, exercise history, and genetics have been factored into the way your body operates today. Learn how your body parts interact with each other. When something hurts, stretch or make adjustments before you accommodate your body around the pain. Oftentimes that accommodation just moves the problem, causing pain to pop up somewhere else.

Your body craves balance. For that reason, when you begin to feel this system augment your well-being, you will have moments when you feel lighter on your feet and more in tune with your body. Those moments last longer as the significance of what you're learning really sinks in. The more you learn, the greater will be your knowledge and control of your body, so that you can walk yourself well with every step you take.

NECK PAIN: CARL

The side of Carl's neck felt like it was being squeezed in a clamp.

Carl's neck hurt constantly, right at the base and to the side a bit. Relaxation and aspirin helped for a while. But even after a weekend of rest and the strongest over-the-counter pain relievers, the side of his neck felt like it was being squeezed by a clamp.

Carl, a newspaper journalist, was thirty-two years old. He didn't like to exercise, and he didn't participate in sports. He was one of those people who shunned physical activity in favor of mental activity. He was extremely articulate, well-mannered, intelligent, and a talented musician.

I learned that Carl had had asthma as a kid, which might have explained why he was never big on sports. But there was more. He had extremely pronated feet and knock-knees. His neck was too long. He wore huge black glasses that were always sliding down his nose. Carl never did anything really physical by nature, so he couldn't figure out what he'd done to cause all the pain. He didn't even *watch* sports, much less participate in them, so the source of his pain became a frustrating mystery. He finally went to his family doctor.

The chain of unsuccessful treatments began with an orthopedic specialist who prescribed muscle relaxants and anti-inflammatories. Carl was also given a booklet with some neck exercises and was told to use them to reduce stress. He tried the neck exercises and started going to a gym three times a week. Carl hadn't been to a gym since junior high, and he hated the concept. But he went anyway.

The drugs reduced the pain, which allowed him to function at work, but there was always a lingering ache that worsened as the day progressed. He did the neck stretches and exercised regularly. His frustration mounted.

Ironically, Carl's trips to the gym were his downfall. He was lifting too much weight and exercising within the parameters of his old Primary Movement Pattern. In addition to the characteristics identified earlier, he had a severely forward head and a rounded upper back. He also took short, shallow breaths up into his chest (habits learned from childhood asthma), and he leaned back when he walked. By working out in his old patterns he was actually making those patterns stronger, thus worsening his condition.

Normally, the factors that cause structural weakness start at your feet and move up. In Carl's case, his asymmetries started at the top and worked down. Carl had a long neck and his glasses slipped a lot, so he kept holding his head in odd positions in an attempt to keep them on. He loved to write, but as he did, he leaned forward. He also played the flute, which put additional strain on his neck.

To hold up his head, his shoulders had to come to the rescue, which caused his upper back to be rounded. This caused a forward inclination from his shoulders to his head, which was counterbalanced as the rest of his body leaned back. Because his center of gravity was to the rear, he locked his knees and rolled his feet to maintain balance. That scenario produced a weak neck, exacerbated by his loves of writing and playing the flute (a vicious circle).

This weak Primary Movement Pattern left Carl with a vulnerable neck that might have caused problems far beyond pain. If he had been in a car accident, it might have had more damaging effects. For example, whiplash can take years to heal when compounded by an acute preexisting weakness.

We started to unravel Carl's asymmetries from the floor up by depronating his feet. We accomplished that through strengthening exercises like the Alphabet. When he learned to open his knees slightly (headlight knees), they automatically unlocked, which made it easy to get his body up and over. He used the Groucho Marx exercise to strengthen his ankles, knees, hips, and belly, and he could do the Tiptoes exercise while dressing in the morning.

He did Side-Lying Neck Rotations, Neck Extensions, and the Cross Crawl to prepare for his gym workout, which he changed to include lots of Press-ups for upper back flexibility. He increased his stamina using a treadmill, with which he simultaneously practiced his new gait. His head moved back to where it belonged, directly above his shoulders, not out in front. His upper back, abs, and neck muscles became strong, and he locked in all his gait corrections. And he had no more pain.

Now Carl writes more prolifically than ever. He is a happy, nimble, pain-free flautist, and—get this—he not only enjoys working out at the gym, he joined a company softball team!

Carl's Personal Profile	Carl's Gait Corrections	His Exercises
outside heel strike, pronated feet	pull heels out, widen stance, open knees,	Alphabet, Tiptoes, Dial Outs, Side-Lying Straight Leg Raises, Calf Stretch on Wall
locked knees	unlock knees, open knees	Knee Extensions, Groucho Marx, Standing Sartorius
sits in hips, tight hip flexors	lift, up and over	Hip Extensions, Hip Flexor Stretch
walks leaning back	lift, up and over	Belly Press, Sitting Hip Flexors, Alternating Knees, Double Knees, Cross Crawl, Supine Stretch Routine
breathes straight up	breathe sideways	Belly Press with Sideways Breathing
round upper back	pull chin in, shoulders and chest down	Modified Push-ups, Sitting Lats, Press-ups
forward head	pull head up and back	Neck Flexors, Neck Extensions, Side-Lying Neck Rotations, Seated Back and Neck Stretch with Shoulder Rolls

NECK PAIN: KARI

The pain in the side of her neck had no pattern. No single thing appeared to start it, and no single thing made it go away.

The left side of Kari's neck felt like an ice pick was sticking into it. She said that her pain came and went and that it had no pattern. There was nothing that always brought it on, and certainly nothing that guaranteed that it would go away. Sometimes she woke up in agonizing pain, and sometimes her nights were peaceful. Sometimes it got worse in the middle of the day, and then days would go by without a chirp of pain.

In Kari's mind, her pain was due to a mild case of scoliosis she'd had since childhood. Scoliosis is a sideways S curve of the spine that can range in seriousness from barely discernible to extreme. It's so common that they test for it in most grade schools, but they often fail to take any remedial steps on the mild cases. Rarely is surgery indicated.

In Kari's parents' minds, Kari was physically limited due to her scoliosis. So they steered her away from sports and toward art. She turned out to be an extremely gifted jewelry designer. Kari didn't miss athletic endeavors, and she didn't really think of herself as being physically weak, either. She was elegant and thin, with long arms and legs, and had blond hair down to her waist. Nobody, including Kari, could see how weak she was.

Kari had a high threshold for pain (she was not a complainer). As a kid she held her back stiff, like a board, to hide the fact that she had a back problem. She walked around as if she had a rod in her back keeping her straight. (Incidentally, that's the surgical treatment for severe scoliosis; they insert a metal rod into the spine.) She thought she could hide the problem. I never did determine whether it was her structural deformity that started the chain of events that culminated in her neck pain or if it was her mental paralysis and subsequent physical paralysis that was the culprit.

Her twin toddlers kept her busy. She had an iron will that allowed her to ignore the neck pain and remain active. Her pain actually disappeared on occasion. But sometimes it nagged at her without a break. On those days even the anti-inflammatories didn't work, and then she'd snap at the kids and feel poorly about everything.

The tension she carried around in her neck was not emotionally based, however, as is often the case. Hers was a physical tension caused by leaning back. She sat in her hips, locked her knees, and had almost no abdominal strength. Although thin, her belly popped out and appeared full. She had no trunk rotation and breathed straight up, so her shoulders rose with each inhale. Most important, her sense of aesthetics didn't allow her to surrender to a forward head, typical of someone with her Primary Movement Pattern. So she had trained herself to use her neck muscles to keep her head up and back all the time, unaware of the damage she was causing. Eventually her little neck just gave in (she put tremendous strain on her sternocleidomastoid muscles, especially on the right side).

After we centered her heel strike and depronated her feet using Fish Feet and Dial Outs, we softened her knees and got them turned out again. The hardest thing for Kari was getting her hip flexors stretched back to normal. She did lots of Table and Double Knees exercises (followed by Hip Flexor Stretches) and finally got that belly tightened. She couldn't have done that without the Belly Press with Sideways Breathing, which enabled her to stay forward on her feet even as she inhaled.

The Supine Stretch Routine helped stretch her lower back, and the Clock Stretch helped her flexibility for trunk rotation. By the time we got to her neck, the pain had already started to subside a little. She used the Seated Back and Neck Stretch with Shoulder Rolls, though she started up on pillows and with really small movements at first. She graduated to Side-Lying Neck Rotations and got to where she could go the full range in a few months. It was just about then that her neck pain turned from chronic to scarce, and even then she had an answer. If she worked long hours on a project and got a little sore, she knew just what to do to stay stretched and strong in all the right places.

Kari's Personal Profile	Kari's Gait Corrections	Her Exercises
outside heel strike, pronated feet, worse on right side	widen stance, leave heels down longer, open knees	Fish Feet, Side-Lying Leg Raises and Hip Circles, Dial Outs, Calf Stretch on Wall
locked knees that turn in, worse on the right side	unlock knees, open knees	Knee Extensions, Semistraight Leg Raises, Standing Sartorius
sits in hips, big lumbar curve, belly pops out	lift, up and over	Upper Ab Crunches, Cross Crawl, Double Knees to Toes, Table Exercise, Hip Flexor Stretch
no trunk rotation	twist body to face each step forward	Sitting Lats, Modified Pushups, Oblique Crunches, Clock Stretch
breathes straight up	breathe sideways	Belly Press with Sideways Breathing
head not forward, but neck and head tense	pull chin and shoulders down, pull head up and back	Side-Lying Neck Rotations, Seated Back and Neck Stretch with Shoulder Rolls

SHOULDER PAIN: REBECCA

Rebecca's shoulder pain was more debilitating than most because it almost cost her the dream of a lifetime.

At twenty-six years of age, Rebecca watched her childhood dream come within reach and then almost slip away. She was offered a spot in the Los Angeles Symphony Orchestra, something she had aspired to all of her life. But something terrible was in the way.

Violinists use the bow to play their instruments, with their arms raised as high as 90 degrees. A lot of shoulder movement takes place as they bow across and back at all sorts of attack angles. But playing a violin for twenty years does very little to balance a Primary Movement Pattern. Especially when you've fashioned yourself after the most endearing musician of all—Mom. Rebecca's mom never had a shoulder problem because she was a pianist. However, she did have a rounded upper back and minor neck pain. Rebecca's body was out of balance to the rear, and the resulting weak link that suffered most was, of course, her shoulder.

Rebecca was totally committed to succeeding as a violinist, so she went to a doctor who gave her anti-inflammatories. She even had a cortisone injection into her biceps tendon. She tried acupuncturists and chiropractors. She tried vacations and rest, and she did the strengthening and stretching work that was prescribed to her by specialists. She ate high-mineral foods for healing and drank lots of water to flush away the inflammation. Most of these remedies produced good results, and some seemed to fix her problem for a while, but none of them kept the pain from returning for good. Rebecca would be playing along perfectly, captured in a world of beautiful music, and then she'd be rudely spun off into horrible pain.

Rebecca played the violin within the parameters of her overall movement pattern—specifically, that of walking. It might be difficult to follow how Rebecca's violin playing was affected by an imbalanced gait, but it was. When some part of your body is out of balance, muscles, ligaments, tendons, and joints tend to be either underworked or overworked. The division of labor is upset. That leads to an eventual vulnerability somewhere, which in Rebecca's case happened to be in the part of her body she moved most often and with the most vigor, her shoulder. So how did the way she walk trickle that far up?

Rebecca had extremely high arches, along with an exaggerated foot-and-hip turnout. When she walked, both heels touched her midline, resulting in a very narrow base of support. She had no calves whatsoever, her knees locked, and she sat in her hips. She had a rounded upper back, and her head and shoulders were forward. That made her shoulder muscles adaptively too short on the front side, so when she drew her bow back, she overstretched that shortened tissue.

We centered her heel strike, pulled her heels out, brought her up and over, and then put her through a rigorous program of strengthening and stretching exercises. Now Rebecca sits in the orchestra without fear that pain will make a rude surprise attack. That's helped her concentration and overall performance. There's nothing like looking back on pain and knowing you've gained the ultimate edge on its ability to intrude.

Rebecca's Personal Profile	Rebecca's Gait Corrections	Her Exercises
huge foot and hip turnout, narrow base of support	widen stance, pull heels out	Dial Outs, Side-Lying Straight Leg Raises
skinny calves	leave heels down longer, lengthen stride	Tiptoes, Wall Stretch Routine
locked knees that turn out	unlock knees	Knee Extensions, Half-moons
sits in hips, leans back, pops belly out	lift, up and over, bring weight forward, twist to face steps	Upper Ab Crunches, Oblique Crunches, Slo-Mo Walking, Hand and Knees Balance, Supine Stretch Routine
round upper back	pull chest and shoulders down	Opposite Arm and Leg, Press-ups, Sitting Lats
forward head and shoulders	pull head up and back, thumbs to front, equalize arm swing	Neck Flexors, Neck Extensions, Side-Lying Neck Rotations, Modified Push-ups, Scapular Push-ups

UPPER BACK AND SHOULDER PAIN: LEONARD

When the pain moved from his right shoulder blade to his left, that bothered him, but when it started to spread across his entire upper back, he panicked.

Leonard's pain started under his right shoulder blade. It was just a nagging ache. It felt a little better after his morning jog, but he began wondering if the doctors were missing something when the pain began to spread. His pain moved from his right shoulder blade to his left and all across his entire upper back. He began to fear that something terrible was going on inside him, and then things got worse. He started losing his range of motion. Leonard started having trouble just pulling a T-shirt over his head, and he began to panic.

At age twenty-eight, Leonard was in good shape and had been physically fit all his life. He'd played varsity tennis in high school and was a distance runner in college. Leonard was a wildly successful import/export entrepreneur who flew overseas every other week. Despite his physical conditioning, and the upgrades to first-class, he still walked off the plane as if he were made of ice-cream sticks, ready to snap any minute.

When I first met Leonard, I saw that he depended heavily on his hip joints to support his weight. He appeared to be in great shape, but his back was somewhat rounded, sort of like you see on a lot of older folks, which is called a kyphotic spine. Upon closer examination I could tell that his forward lean was just a compensation for a center of gravity that had been displaced to the rear. Leonard needed some basic primary movement adjusting.

Leonard told me that as a kid he had had tendonitis in his right shoulder and elbow. He said that he'd missed a few tennis tournaments due to tendonitis when he was a teenager. But getting this information out of him was difficult. I'm not sure if it was pride, cultural background, or his emotionally private nature, but Leonard bottled up his pain and his fears. He wanted to keep them a secret, at least until now.

He told me that he just smiled at his business partners through the pain. He had never complained to his wife. He could barely open up to me. It was clear that he stuffed all his feelings deep inside and they were surfacing internally—fear, fatigue, and even excitement can manifest in the form of physical tension that torques otherwise normal body parts. I convinced Leonard to approach his gait corrections and exercises as an escape program that would lead to mental and physical wellness. He accepted the suggestion.

Here's a partial list of what we needed to work on regarding his Primary Movement Pattern. Leonard had an exaggerated outside heel strike that forced him to sit way back in his hips. His knees locked with each step, and he carried his chest, ribs, and chin high. This all caused his shoulder blades to pull up and back while his shoulders rolled forward. When he walked, the backs of his hands led the way.

We worked especially hard on stretching Leonard's hip flexors and strengthening his lower back and abs so he could stand without sitting way back in his hips. We centered his heel strike by widening his step, which made it possible for him to stop locking his knees. That was a big help in getting Leonard to stay up and over his feet. Leonard did a lot of upper back strengthening, too, using the Opposite Arm and Leg exercise and the Hands and Knees Balance. That helped strengthen his sandwich system which he also needed.

He did Press-ups with a passion to make his upper back flexible, and Scapular Push-ups to strengthen his shoulders and chest. We worked on his forward shoulder roll and his forward head using the Pec Stretch in a Doorjamb stretching exercise, as well as Back Shoulder Rolls and Sitting Lats. He straightened out his arms so his thumbs led the way, which finished the process. Leonard's dedication paid off: his shoulder and upper back pain disappeared.

Although Leonard's kyphotic (curved) upper back didn't vanish, his balanced gait ensures that it's not going to get worse. Those fifteen hour plane trips are still no picnic, but he knows how to stretch and strengthen, and in what position to carry his body, so that every day is a building exercise of painless motion.

Leonard's Personal Profile	Leonard's Gait Corrections	His Exercises
extreme outside heel strike, foot flop	widen stance, hold toes up longer	Alphabet, Side-Lying Straight Leg Raises, Standing Balance, Toes Feet/Feet Toes
locked knees	unlock knees	Knee Extensions, Modified Mini-Squats
sits in hips, tight hip flexors, pops belly out	lift up and over, lengthen steps	Upper Ab Crunches, Double Knees to Toes, Hip Extensions, Hip Flexor Stretch, Supine Stretch Routine
chest, chin, shoulders all very high (military style)	pull chest and shoulders down	Sitting Lats, Modified Push-ups, Scapular Push-ups
round upper back	thumbs to front, breathe sideways	Belly Press, Back Shoulder Rolls
head way forward	pull head up and back	Neck Flexors, Neck Extensions, Side-Lying Neck Rotations

UPPER BACK AND SHOULDER PAIN: SEAN

The pain in Sean's upper back came on slowly, and once it set in, it lingered with an irritable ache all day.

Sean was forty-eight years old when he finally had to ask himself to choose. The big question was which part of his life would he have to give up due to his shoulder and upper back pain: dentistry (his vocation), photography (his passion), or camping (he and his kids loved to camp)? Was it asking too much to have it all, free of pain? Sean was about to give up.

Ever watch how your dentist positions himself as he works on your mouth? They've made progress with the chairs, and they even teach new biotechnically sound approaches, but Sean used the old bend-over-the-patient method, which helped me understand part of his problem. Then there was carrying camping gear and an occasional piggyback ride the last hundred yards out of the woods, not to mention the photographic equipment and lengthy photo shoots.

At first, Sean dealt with his pain by sacrificing his dental practice. He scheduled breaks between patients. He limited his photography to tripod work, and he even found himself a little short-fused with the kids while on shortened hiking trips. An oral hygienist at the office told him about me.

How his activities influenced his Primary Movement Pattern was fascinating. I couldn't tell if Sean's asymmetries had caused the pain (if he was crooked to begin with and his activities of choice intensified his crookedness and caused pain) or if his activities of lifting, twisting, and bending ultimately caused his asymmetries. Most of the time it's the asymmetries that create vulnerabilities, and given the right incident, the weakest link ruptures into actual pain. Either way, it didn't matter. His Primary Movement Pattern was not symmetrical. That I can work with, regardless of whether the egg came before the chicken. The treatment is the same—identify the problematic movement pattern, work in the right gait corrections, back them up with exercises and stretching, and voilà. Not exactly. I wish it was that easy. Unfortunately, it takes focus and work. And that's what he did.

First, my analysis of his Primary Movement Pattern quickly uncovered that his left foot crossed over his midline with way too much turnout. That caused his left shoulder to drop. Try it. Step in with your left foot as you walk and cross over your midline with your toes turned out and watch what happens to your left shoulder. Down it goes. He couldn't recall a childhood injury that could have caused it, but the result was a pretty desperate Primary Movement Pattern.

Sean also had an outside heel strike, worse on the left, and a major pronation as a result. Because his left leg crossed over to the right side, he locked his knee, sat in his hips, leaned back, and then with every left arm swing back, down went the shoulder. His upper body rotation was way too bouncy, up and down, and not horizontal, as it should be. Plus, he carried his head too far forward.

Centering Sean's heel strike on both sides, widening his stance, and pulling his heels out just about fixed his entire gait. Amazing! I watched his feet move into position, and his upper body balanced itself immediately. He came up and over on his feet and began rotating his shoulders horizontally.

We had to work on his left shoulder dropping to the rear as a separate item. (I imagined the hours and hours he'd spent twisted slightly to the right with his left arm up and his shoulder blade pulled back, peering into mouth after mouth.) To do that, I asked him to lead with his left pinky finger on his arm swing back and at the same time to exaggerate the forward motion of his right shoulder. That kept his left shoulder in place. But it wasn't easy. That deeply ingrained habit was hard to break.

Sean still prefers dentistry the old-fashioned way. He twists freely with his camera to get any angle he feels like. And best of all, he's an all-around happy camper.

Sean's Personal Profile	Sean's Gait Corrections	His Exercises
outside heel strike and foot turnout, worse on left, foot pronation	widen stance, pull heels out, open knees	Side-Lying Straight Leg Raises and Hip Circles, Dial Outs, Fish Feet, Towel Scrunches, Standing Sartorius
locked knees	unlock knees	Knee Extensions, Modified Mini-Squats

Sean's Personal Profile	Sean's Gait Corrections	His Exercises
sits in hips, leans back	lift up and over	Upper Ab Crunches, Cross Crawl, Hands and Knees Balance, Supine Stretch Routine
left arm drops down and back	equalize arm swings, thumbs to front	Sitting Lats, Modified Push-ups, Scapular Push-ups, Clock Stretch
head forward	pull head up and back	Neck Flexors, Neck Extensions, Seated Back and Neck Stretch with Shoulder Rolls

LOWER BACK PAIN: ROY

Roy had two ruptured disks and was in so much pain he couldn't move. But surgery was not an option for him.

Some patients are in such a calamitous condition that they can't come to me; I have to go to them. Roy's pain was critical. It emanated from his lower back. He hurt from his right bun all the way down his thigh to his heel. But the focus of his anguish was directly in the middle of his lower back. Roy had two ruptured disks. Several top-notch doctors had come up with the same diagnosis, and they each indicated that surgery was his best alternative.

Roy loathed the concept of isolating himself in a hospital for weeks, of having doctors cut him open, and of accepting a serious operation with no guarantees. Roy had lots of initiative, and all his life had been driven to pursue physical fitness. He was an avid golfer and sports enthusiast. He strived for the healthiest, strongest body possible, and since he'd been committed to that quest for years, he saw no reason to give in to surgery now. So Roy chose his own defense plan.

Roy fully believed that if he stayed off his feet, those two damaged disks would manage to repair themselves. He felt that that meant bed rest, mainly because moving was so painful. So he created a little universe around his bedroom, including office space, a mini-kitchen, a water supply, reading material, and even a play area for the kids. The most impressive thing he brought to that room, however, was the will to stick it out. (Roy didn't like staying still for long.)

Weeks went by, and he remained convinced that healing himself was just a matter of time and rest. His doctors didn't agree, but one doctor told him if he was going to continue pursuing that strategy he'd need a physical therapist to stretch and strengthen the rest of his body while his back got well, assuming it was getting well at all. Everybody agreed on the need for physical therapy.

Since he was not up and walking around, I had no clue what his Primary Movement Pattern looked like. He told me he'd broken his right hip falling off a horse when he was ten years old, but besides that, all I knew was that spending so much time in bed must have sapped his strength. It had. He was also in almost constant pain. The pain was so bad that turning over nearly made him break into tears.

My experience with Dr. McKenzie's theories gave me an edge in working with Roy's pain, which is what I wanted to deal with first. The exercise he needed most required that he be on his stomach, but it was so painful for him to get to that position that we needed to begin with the most basic of all moves, belly tightening. By teaching him how to tighten in preparation for turning, he was able to get into the position to do Press-ups, which are designed to deal with his type of back condition and weakness. Unfortunately, he barely had the arm strength to do the Press-ups. But his tenacity indicated that he'd be a good candidate for homework assignments. So I left him with strengthening work to do on his own and an explanation of how vital each and every repetition was to him.

By the second visit he was a little more malleable, and the belly tightening and the Press-ups had decreased his pain—not a lot, but any sign was a good one at that point. By the third visit he was actually sitting on the edge of the bed, which might not sound like much, but getting there was important for adding additional exercises.

In the beginning he could sit up for only short periods before the pain drove him back down again. When he did sit up, I could see that his idea of posture was not good. That was part of the reason he couldn't sit up very long. His posture induced spasms and pain. (He didn't know that sitting up high, with his back arched and his chest puffed out, was just as bad as slouching, and maybe worse.) I showed him how to soften and come down a bit to reduce his postural rigidity and get more out of his belly strength.

Soon he was able to approach the monumental task of getting to his feet. To accomplish this, I showed him how to widen his stance, to use his hands to push himself up and onto the balls of his feet, and to keep his belly tight, chin down, and buns underneath him. Standing up delighted him, but every time he tried to walk, his pain returned, so he'd go back to bed and assume the fetal position, which reduced his suffering.

Despite his agony, those brief little walks really paid off, because I could see what his Primary Movement Pattern looked like. He had an outside heel strike on the right and not the left, and only his right foot turned out. He had a narrow base of support, but neither foot crossed over his midline. He locked both knees. His right hip punched way out at mid-stance (right side), and he had weak lower abs. (He was a little embarrassed to learn that all the ab work he'd done had worked only on his upper abs. He had unknowingly neglected the lowers.) He had no trunk rotation (he carried his body as if it were a cement block). And, as you may have suspected, he sat in his hips and leaned back when he walked. The good news was that I understood his Primary Movement Pattern, so I could map out a program to begin his recovery.

Roy started with Alphabet and Fish Feet exercises while lying on his back, knees up, one foot at a time. He'd cross one foot over his

Roy's Personal Profile	Roy's Gait Corrections	His Exercises
outside heel strike and foot turnout, right side	pull heels out, especially the right	Alphabet, Fish Feet, Dial Outs, Side-Lying Straight Leg Raises, and Hip Circles
locked knees	unlock knees	Knee Extensions (one at a time)
right hip punch	widen left step	Inner Thighs, Wall Stretch Routine, Hands and Knees Balance
sits in hips, buns tucked way under, weak lower abs	lift up and over	Opposite Arm and Leg, Hip Extensions, Half-moons, Table Exercise, Alternating Knees, Double Knees to Toes, Supine Stretch Routine
no trunk rotation	twist the torso, open the knees	Clock Stretch, Standing Sartorious
head slightly forward	pull head up and back	Neck Extensions

other knee to get his foot in the air. He needed to rebuild ab strength, but Belly Presses (the most direct route) would have put downward pressure on his spine, which might compress the sciatic nerve, which could intensify his leg pain. So we worked on his abs indirectly by having him do Side-Lying Straight Leg Raises and Hip Circles, which he needed anyway to eliminate the hip punch.

Once he was able to sit up to do Dial Outs and Sitting Hip Flexors, he improved rapidly. He could even walk around the house several times before the pain came back. But the most inspiring pain breakthrough occurred in conjunction with the Supine Stretch Routine. It worked like magic. Because he experienced pain relief when he crossed his foot over to the other knee, I could tell that his leg pain was caused by a tight piriformis muscle (the one that turns the hip out, which was part of why his hip punched out).

With every visit I added more exercises. He did Half-moons for strengthening his hips, Hip Extension over Pillows, and Hands and Knees Balance for back and belly strength. Finally the day came for a walk outside. He could manage a full ten minutes, and then he had to plop down on someone's lawn and spend a moment restretching his piriformis. If someone walked by, Roy just froze and pretended to be a lawn jockey. The walks did wonders for Roy, and he made steady progress (with a few exceptions—like the time he went to the driving range a little prematurely).

After a few months, Roy was doing Belly Presses, the Cross Crawl, Alternating Knees, and lots of Press-ups in between. Roy conquered his back problem without surgery and returned to a normal life shortly thereafter. He still does ab and hip exercises, and he appreciates golf more than ever.

LOWER BACK PAIN: MS. LEVY

Ms. Levy had a good spirit and a bad back that left her stranded on the floor waiting for help.

Ms. Levy hobbled into my office with a slow trickle of unstoppable tears. She was experiencing intolerable pain in her lower back and left buttock. She was certain she needed a massage, or a few massages, to make the world right again. Then she found out what we do in my office. She wasn't amused. She didn't want to be marched around in an attempt to learn a new way to walk. She really wanted a massage. She wasn't getting one. More tears.

Ms. Levy's orthopedic doctor had sent her directly to me. Good thing, too, because delaying her recovery might have led to surgery. She had a large protruding disk that showed its ugly face on the MRI scan. So we weren't going to dally around with a warm fuzzy massage, which in this case would only serve as a Band-Aid, and might have taken away from the time we needed to really correct her problem.

Ms. Levy was a grade school teacher, and had been for years. She taught art, and she frequently lugged around a huge box of art supplies. When she first lifted the box out of her trunk one morning, her back twinged. Then she stopped to chat with two children in the playground with the box resting on her left hip. Her back twinged again.

When she got to class, she hoisted the box up onto a shelf, and her final twinge left her on her back and staring at the ceiling. There she stayed, on the floor, waiting for the bell to ring so the doors would open and someone would find her and bring help. That help turned out to be her doctor, who, along with some other orthopedic and neurologic doctors, knew that even large disk problems can often be "fixed" without surgery.

So Ms. Levy went through the gait correction and exercise routine, kicking and screaming for the first few sessions. She continued only because we promised her that when she got the basic concepts down and at least knew what a balanced gait looked like, she could negotiate for a massage once a week. But first she needed to understand that we were attempting to heal her thoroughly and that a massage would not do that. She understood, and she still wanted that massage so badly she paid perfect attention. In fact, she totally restructured how she walked and moved. Good thing, too, because Ms. Levy had quite a few problems going on.

Ms. Levy was built solidly, with a big belly, a big back, a barrel chest, and the most tucked-under buns I'd ever seen. I found out the reason later. Up until a few years earlier, Ms. Levy had been an aerobics class junkie. She did millions of those old-time donkey kicks, which give you strange heart-shaped buns, tight at the top and outsides but floppy at the bottom. Anyway, during that time she was always able to do twice as many of those kick things on the right as on the left. Her left hip always felt weaker. And she had always been taught to tuck her buns under. She also had been indoctrinated to think that sitting up straight, way too straight, was a good thing.

As for her personal movement profile, she had an outside heel strike, her left foot pronated and crossed over her midline, and it turned way out. Her knees locked and pointed inward (that was an uncommon one, to have a turned-out foot and a turned-in knee, but it happens). She had skinny inner calves and large outer calves. She sat in her hips, and her right hip pooched out. She leaned back a lot, breathed straight upward, and had a forward head (and a double chin).

Strengthening and balancing Ms. Levy's hips practically set her entire movement pattern in order. First we had to fix her sartorius muscle to get rid of that pronation, foot turnout, and knee locking. She supplemented the gait corrections with the Alphabet exercise, which she did in calligraphy (being an art teacher), and she walked on her toes a lot to even out her calves (she even did that with a wide right step to neutralize her left hip punch).

She had to do a lot of Hip Extensions (which she did in all three positions) to balance the strength of her buttocks (her top part was too strong). Learning to breathe sideways was not easy for her, and the belly work was difficult, too, since it meant breaking some deeply ingrained patterns. The last step was to work on her neck. We moved her head back to where it was supposed to be and arranged for her to have her blessed massage. It turned out to be a clear case of win-win therapy.

Ms. Levy's Personal Profile	Ms. Levy's Gait Corrections	Her Exercises
outside heel strike, left foot pronated, crosses midline, huge foot turnout	heel strike on inside, open knees, widen stance, pull heels out	Alphabet, Fish Feet, Standing Sartorius, Side-Lying Straight Leg Raises, Dial Outs, Hip Flexors

Ms. Levy's Personal Profile	Ms. Levy's Gait Corrections	Her Exercises
locked knees, pointed inward	unlock knees, headlight knees (beams out)	Knee Extensions, more Standing Sartorius
skinny inner calves	lengthen steps, leave heels down longer	Tiptoes, Hip Extensions, Wall Stretch Routine, Hip Flexor Stretch
sits in hips and leans back, left hip pooched out	up and over, trunk twist, widen right step	Hip Slider Reaches, Alternating Knees, Double Knees to Toes, lots of Press-ups, Inner Thighs 2 Ways
breathes straight up, barrel-chested	breathe sideways	Belly Press with sideways breath, Sitting Lats, Modified Push-ups, Scapular Push-ups
forward head and double chin	pull head up and back, pull chest and shoulders down	Neck Flexors, Neck Extensions, Sitting Lats, Standing Back Bends

HIP PAIN: LENA

It felt like someone was driving a sharp nail straight into the back of her hip socket.

Lena held on to her appealing personality as she waddled into my office in pain. Pregnancy is formidable enough without the exasperation of interim pain. I admired her spirit as she explained that she felt like someone was driving a nail straight into the back of her hip socket. It was driving her bonkers.

While sitting there, Lena turned from completely composed to seriously melancholy, to absolutely forlorn. With a misty glance she confessed that the pain had made her lose composure in the kitchen earlier that week. She said that the other day she'd helped her husband off to work, smiling as best she could to cover up her painful hip. But after he'd driven off, she staggered back to the kitchen and hurled two dishes at the wall. I told her that her experiment proved beyond any doubt that dishes make incredibly bad Frisbees, and with a grin and a Kleenex we proceeded to collect data on her real problem.

The pain began a few months into her pregnancy, but because it hurt less sometimes than at other times, she didn't pay much attention to it. She was convinced that it was the baby pushing on some nerve that was connected to her hip and that there wasn't much she could do about it. Still, she felt trapped, and having so much to accomplish, from preparing the baby's room to running her graphic design business, she was not coping well. A friend of hers finally dragged her to my office door.

I learned that her pain was worse later in the day, almost always pursuant to certain activities: driving, going to the theater, eating at restaurants, doing computer work. In other words, sitting. There was no real connection between increased pain and walking. I also learned that the only way she found relief was to lie on the couch on her right side, leaning against the back of the couch (that's the only way she could see the TV). She didn't know that by lying on her right side she was helping to put her lower back and hips into line with her spine, thus centralizing her torso. All she knew was that it reduced her pain.

The day she arrived in my office she hadn't been sitting long enough for her to start the cycle of hip pain, so she could walk comfortably as I watched. Lena was five feet, eight inches tall and a natural beauty, with dark skin, big green eyes, and the sinewy body of a model. I learned shortly thereafter that she *was* a model and that she was in terrific shape partially as the result of her cardiovascular work, which she divided among an exercise bike, a stair-stepper, and a treadmill. She felt confident that her pain had nothing to do with physical weakness. Indeed, before her pregnancy she'd looked strong, felt strong, and had experienced no pain at all.

Her Primary Movement Pattern revealed the entire story, and the puzzle clicked into place immediately. Her right foot had a distinct outside heel strike and an exaggerated turnout (her left foot was okay). When she walked, her right foot actually crossed over her midline. Her right knee faced out (her left knee faced forward). Her knees locked when she walked, she sat back into her hips, and she punched her right hip way out at mid-stance. It was perfect: she displayed the typical gait of a runway model.

The human body can take abuse for longer periods of time when it's young, flexible, and slender. Lena's exaggerated, slinky gait worked well for her until she added the weight of pregnancy. Without the pregnancy, her structural vulnerabilities might not have surfaced until later in life, but either way, the gait of a runway model is often not structurally sound. It's quite the opposite.

It took a few sessions to get Lena up and over her feet, but after we did, that eliminated the pregnant waddle. Since she was strong and "body aware," she caught on quickly to widening her left foot when she walked to stop her right hip from protruding. Among other gait corrections and exercises, I had her do the Sitting Stretch Routine, the Hands and Knees Balance exercise, the Side-Lying Straight Leg Raises and Hip Circles, and Hip Extensions on Hands and Knees (all safe when pregnant). Once Lena overcame the weakness in her hip and stopped popping it out when she walked, the pain disappeared. The remaining gait corrections fell into place easily, and within six weeks the only pain she had to work through was the glorious pain of delivering her little girl (six pounds, five ounces).

Note for Pregnant Women: Some doctors don't like their pregnant patients to do exercises lying on their backs. That's because they fear cutting off the blood supply to the placenta. Other doctors don't think that's an issue because if that occurred, they'd feel light-headed and sit up immediately, thus eliminating the problem. Either way, don't do exercises lying on your back without your doctor's recom-

Lena's Personal Profile	Lena's Gait Corrections	Her Exercises
big outside heel strike on right (a little on left), big foot turnout on right (a little on left)	heel strike on inside, pull heels out	Alphabet, Fish Feet, Dial Outs
locked knees, right knee points out, left knee points straight ahead	unlock knees, open knees	Modified Mini-Squats, Half-moons, Standing Sartorius
major right hip punch (classic model gait), sits in hips, leans back	widen left step, lift up and over	Inner Thighs, Side-Lying Straight Leg Raises and Hip Circles, Hands and Knees Balance, Wall Stretch Routine
pregnant belly too far out	more lift up and over, breathe sideways, twist torso	Belly Press with sideways breathing, Clock Stretch
forward head	pull head up and back	Neck Extensions

mendation. Lena did lots of exercises in other positions. She did only one exercise on her back—and she had no problems with it.

HIP PAIN: JERRY

The pain was always in one place—at the top front of his hip, just under where you can feel your hipbone stick out. And it hurt with every step.

Jerry's pain was an occasional visitor at first, but it gradually became a full-time resident. His hip really hurt when he walked, and it even bugged him while he was trying to sleep. So he decided to take the athletic stuff down a notch and gave up windsurfing. After that he gave up basketball, and then golf. Soon, the only exercise Jerry permitted himself was working out at the gym, something he felt he had to do just to keep healthy.

Everything seemed to make the pain flair up, which made it difficult to pinpoint exactly what was causing the problem. And to worsen the investigative matter, the pain wouldn't show up until the day following some rigorous activity. Jerry finally resorted to anti-inflammatories as a test, and when that didn't do the trick, he went on to acupuncture, cortisone injections, and therapeutic massages, all of which were very helpful. So he'd go and play basketball again, and the next thing he knew the pain had returned, just as bad as before.

Jerry was an architect who had to stand or sit for mega-hours while drawing. Standing and sitting so much is what gave him all those outside sports cravings. He said they allowed him to "unclog." As a kid Jerry had always been good at sports, and he played them all. His body was in great shape. In fact, at first glance I wondered what in the world could be wrong with this guy.

I spotted a short step on the left, but we'd all take a short step on a side with a painful anything. So I ruled that out temporarily. I noticed a slight left hip hike, though not a big hip punch like I often see with patients with similar hip pain complaints. Jerry did his hip hike at the end of the pushoff on that side. I saw no sign of any back or knee problems, and his gait was amazingly good. He had nice rotation, springy knees, and he didn't even lean back. So I asked him to remove his clothes from the ankle down. With his shoes and socks off I could see his heel strike more clearly.

That's when I noticed that his left big toe didn't bend! Why, I asked, don't you bend your big toe on that side when you walk? He told me that he'd broken it a few years back and hadn't been comfortable bending it ever since. He managed to maintain a perfectly comfortable way to walk, run, jump, golf, surf, and everything else. Only a great athlete could have pulled that off, but he did. The problem was that it couldn't last forever without backfiring. By learning to walk without putting much weight on his toe, he developed an outside heel strike. He also had a quick, jerky way to pick up that foot, which he accomplished quite well with his hip. His quadratus lumborum muscle did most of the work, and as a result, he'd just slightly overstretch the front of that hip with each step.

Getting back to the toe thing, have you tried walking without using your big toes? Go ahead, try it. Only if you're extremely well balanced can you walk like that without developing a multitude of problems, if you can do it at all. Had Jerry gone on like that, his hip wouldn't have been his only trouble. Fortunately, he caught the problem in time.

Jerry actually needed orthotics (shoe inserts made by professionals, or in some cases available off-the-shelf in drugstores) to gently raise his arches and stabilize his feet. He also needed a lot of physical therapy on his toe. Our job was to center his heel strike. We did Toes Feet/Feet Toes until it came out of his ears. He had to be able to put weight on that toe. (Had there been no way to bend the toe, we'd have had to come up with some other fancy shenanigans to rework his hip mechanics into a workable fashion. Fortunately, his toe still bent, though it took time and it hurt a little to get there.)

Muscles weaken quickly with disuse, and although Jerry looked strong (and was strong), certain spots were extremely weak. He needed to do Hip Flexors, Hip Extensors, and Side-Lying Hip Circles to rebalance his weight-bearing superstructure. Jerry was able to restrengthen himself back to peak performance. Now after a tough day at his desk, he goes home and sits quietly by the fire and knits. Of course I'm kidding, he crochets.

Jerry's Personal Profile	Jerry's Gait Corrections	His Exercises
outside heel strike on left	center heel strike	Alphabet, Toes Feet/ Feet Toes
left hip hike, short left step	leave heel down longer, slow down swing phase on right side	Standing Balance, Hip Extensions, Side-Lying Straight Leg Raises and Hip Circles, Slo-Mo Walking, Hip Flexor Stretch, Supine Stretch Routine, Calf Stretch on Wall
left shoulder back	equalize arm swings	Oblique Crunches, Clock Stretch

KNEE PAIN: MATHEW

Knee pain doesn't always stem from weak ankles. Mathew's ankles were healthy. He just demanded too much of them because of the way he walked, and that led to damage and pain elsewhere.

Successful, high-powered lawyers don't need to do yard work, but some still do. Mathew loved scuffing around in the compost because it felt therapeutic. He loved being active in his garden, and he loved gourmet cooking, vintage ports, Stilton cheese, and, well, eating. The catch was that he was about forty pounds overweight and not fond of formal exercise. Gardening was good for him.

I met Mathew after his second knee surgery, not on the same knee. The first knee went out on him when he brought his bicycle to a stop at a corner. He put his leg down for balance and stepped down with a locked knee. Youch. His ligaments didn't do too well, as demonstrated by the swelling, pain, and ensuing surgery three weeks later.

His other knee gave way a year after he'd completed the rehabilitation on his first knee. Only this time the knee injury was caused by slipping on the back porch stairs. The result, however, was the same. His second knee required the same surgery as the first.

His surgery was performed at one of the most prestigious orthopedic hospitals in Los Angeles. Afterward, Mathew was sent to another section of the hospital for clinical rehab work. They strengthened his knee, of course, and slowly worked him back into health. The sad thing was that they didn't take any steps to correct, nor did they even identify, what had caused Mathew's problem in the first place. They didn't see or acknowledge that both of his knees were very hyperextended when he stood or walked. They treated the injured area, but they missed the underlying weakness. Nothing was done to prevent another accident from happening. They treated only the symptom. They missed the cause.

Mathew's Primary Movement Pattern was no big surprise. He practically walked on his inner ankles (his feet were badly pronated). Imagine a big guy to start with, schlepping a fifty-pound roll of sod with locked knees and ankles rolled in. Gnarly. Mathew had a severe inside heel strike, a narrow base of support, and major foot turnout. In addition to pronation and hyperextended knees, he sat back in his hips, leaned back when he walked, had his shoulders and head way forward, and was virtually bereft of abdominal strength. What a target. You might wonder why his back didn't blow out on him. I sure did. But people usually injure their weakest link first, and that link usually has to do with physical dimensions and proportions.

Since Mathew was recovering from knee surgery, we had to stick to the sitting exercises to strengthen his feet and knees. I couldn't wait to get this guy up and doing the Slo-Mo Walking and Groucho Marx exercises, all with soft knees and lots of trunk rotation. After a month of nothing but strengthening, it was great to see how well he was able to execute the standing exercises. We did all the sandwich system work, starting with the Belly Press and going straight on through to the Table Exercise and Double Knees to Toes with weights on. Mathew began his flexibility work with the Seated Back and Neck Stretch, and by the time he left, he was happily on "the wall"! (After five to ten minutes of crouching around doing the Groucho Marx exercise, the wall seemed like a real treat to him.)

I tried to convince Mathew to confront his weight problem, but he wasn't interested in being any smaller. Fortunately, he's much better equipped to carry around that extra weight now, because now he walks with power and balance.

Mathew's Personal Profile	Mathew's Gait Corrections	His Exercises
extreme pronation, extreme foot turnout (heels touch), inside heel strike	widen stance, pull heels out, center heel strike	Alphabet, Fish Feet, Dial Outs, Toes Feet/Feet Toes, Hip Flexor Stretch
locked knees	unlock knees	Semistraight Leg Raises, Knee Extensions, Slo-Mo Walking, Groucho Marx
sits in hips, leans back	up and over	Belly Press, Double Knees to Toes, Seated Back and Neck Stretch, Wall Stretch Routine
forward head and shoulders, breathes up into chest	pull head up and back, breathe sideways	Belly Press with Sideways Breathing, Neck Flexors, Neck Extensors, Sitting Lats, Pec Stretch in and Door Jamb

KNEE PAIN: MEGAN

Megan's knees used to hurt only after some form of strenuous exercise, but soon her knees hurt all the time, even after a long walk.

Under normal circumstances, Megan's right knee might have remained pain-free for years. But Megan was no normal kid. She loved ice-skating, and she had amazing athletic abilities. She was already working on double jumps, and her coach had no problem pacing her aggressively because she was so outrageously talented. The knee problem surfaced when she filled in for the school basketball team. She couldn't resist the offer to play, and that was it for her knee.

After that, any sporting activity made her knees hurt. They even hurt after she sat for a while. When she skated, her right knee would swell a little at the back and on the inside. Jumping was out of the question. Her right leg was her landing leg. After three jumps, she'd swell up so much that even her coach got the message.

Pretty soon her knees hurt all the time, even after just a little walking. When she rested from skating and sports, her right knee stopped swelling and her knees felt okay, but inactivity was no solution. Megan was too spirited and precocious to sit still long, and she decided to ask for help. That was my cue.

Megan had a slight ligament strain. Her drive to skate had probably saved her from future injuries, because without the pain she'd encountered while skating she might have been unaware of her vulnerability and continued to walk herself into deeper problems as the years passed.

Megan was the perfect candidate for a knee injury. She was five feet, three inches tall and built like a toothpick. That part was fine, but her shy personality caused her to curl her upper body forward as if she wanted to wither up whenever she wasn't participating in sports. So her upper back was rounded forward and her head was too far forward, too. She had an outside heel strike and too much turnout on both feet. She sat in her hips and leaned back.

I got to watch Megan skate, which was simply amazing. On the ice, all her gait deviations went away. Her body was perfectly balanced, torso up and over, looking good. Her head was a little too far forward, especially when she did a spiral, which is when a leg goes way up in back and you glide for a long time, and her shoulders needed to stay down a tad, but otherwise she was a graceful beauty. That is, until she took off her skates. That's when the "shy teenager" walk, which obliterated her instinctual balance on the ice, returned.

We started with Alphabets and Towel Scrunches for her feet. For her knees she did Semistraight Leg Raises, Modified Mini-Squats (very tiny ones to start), and Knee Extensions. She also used a mini-trampoline (starting with a million tiny little jumps), which had the added benefit of developing the muscles she needed to jump for skating. She used Hip Flexors and Dial Outs, the Table Exercise, and Double Knees to Toes to stop her from leaning back. Although her head used to stick out too far forward, Megan didn't need neck work because she hadn't spent that many years locking in her improper head carriage. As soon as she stopped leaning back, her head popped right back up to where it belonged.

Megan's Personal Profile	Megan's Gait Corrections	Her Exercises
outside heel strike, extreme foot turnout	center heel strike, pull heels out	Alphabet, Dial Outs, Towel Scrunches, Hip Flexor Stretch
locked knees	unlock knees	Semistraight Leg Raises, Modified Mini-Squats, Knee Extensions, use of a mini-trampoline
sits in hips	lift up and over	Hands and Knees Balance, Opposite Arm and Leg, Double Knees to Toes, Table Exercise
forward head and shoulders	pull head up and back	Neck Flexors, Neck Extensions, Sitting Lats, Press-ups, Standing Back Bends

ANKLE PAIN: GREG

Greg was actually embarrassed to go to the doctor with a sprained ankle. It just didn't seem serious enough to warrant medical attention. But the pain didn't go away, so he sought help.

Greg was twenty-eight years old and a firefighter. He'd hurt his ankle during a fire as he descended some stairs in a rush. The surprising part was that he hadn't hurt one of his ankles sooner. He was basically an accident waiting to happen.

Greg's doctor told him he had sustained a stress injury in his ankle and put him in a walking cast for six weeks. That dealt with his immediate problem. Fortunately, he was also put into physical therapy for modalities (that's cold packs, ultrasound, electric stimulation, and strengthening exercise), too. That gave me the opportunity to work on the underlying source of his problem to prevent it from happening again.

Both of his feet had really high arches, which usually means there won't be a problem with foot pronation. But his feet were pronated. When I examined his foot, it looked swollen at the inner ankle bone. It turned out that some of what appeared to be swelling was actually a shift in the bones toward the center at his ankle; it wasn't swelling at all. The bone shift was due to his pronation.

All of Greg's gait deviations were actually pretty minor. That is, he had his share, but no single deviation was all that exaggerated. Greg had an outside heel strike, a little too much foot turnout, and a narrow base of support. He sat in his hips, had a slight forward head, and no trunk rotation to speak of. The most glaring problem he had was in his feet. His extremely high arches caused most, if not all, of his gait deviations and ankle problems.

Greg's ankles might have been imposed upon him genetically, but had he learned the concept of getting up and over on his feet earlier in life, he might have avoided his current situation. Because he was so tall and solid, his arches were bound to cause him problems. Those problems developed into a stress injury. (The force on your feet and arches increases significantly as your activity level goes up, and that additional force increases the liklihood of stress-related injuries.)

We centered his heel strike using Fish Feet and Dial Outs. And we got him some arch supports to put in all his shoes—most important, his work boots. (That way, the floor comes up to meet the foot instead of the foot being forced to meet the floor.) Greg did a lot of foot-strengthening exercises like the Alphabet, Tiptoes, and Toes Feet/Feet Toes. He had a lot of compensating to do for those arches.

He strengthened his upper abs (his lower abs were already quite strong) to reinforce the up-and-over correction. He added Oblique Crunches to his exercise routine to increase trunk rotation. Outer Hip Circles made it easier to widen his base of support. And he did the Wall Stretch Routine, among other things, to stretch his hips so his buns didn't pull back so hard, and to help pull his heels out. So it was back to full-on firefighting for Greg, which is really where he and his ankles wanted to be.

Greg's Personal Profile	Greg's Gait Corrections	His Exercises
pronation, with extremely high arches, outside heel strikes	open knees slightly, center heels	Alphabet, Fish Feet, Toes Feet/Feet Toes, Calf Stretch on Wall
knees pointed straight ahead	open knees slightly	Standing Sartorius, Hip Flexor Stretch
sits in hips, tight lower back, tight hip flexors, big lumbar curve (buns stick out)	lift up and over, leave heels down longer	Double Knees to Toes, Table Exercise, Low Ab Knee Switchers, Hands and Knees Balance, Press-ups, Supine Stretch Routine, Wall Stretch Routine

ANKLE PAIN: ZOEY

Zoey's ankles didn't hurt all the time, but it seemed as if she was constantly reinjuring them.

Zoey had a long history of sprained ankles, the last of which occurred as she stepped out of the shower. Her ankle rolled down, and *boing*, there it went. She'd sprained it again.

This accident came on the same afternoon she finished swimming a twenty-nine-minute mile, which is not bad for a recreational athlete of fifty. She used to play tennis regularly, but running and twisting sports had led to five previous ankle sprains. So she took up swimming as a safe new form of exercise. She grew quite fond of the quiet solitude of the water, and she missed tennis less and less as she gave her ankles a long-needed break. But this sprain that happened as she stepped out of the shower was absolutely mortifying. And it hurt!

Someone referred her to me four weeks after the injury. Her ankle was pitifully weak by then. After treating her with the regular forms of preliminary therapy (ice, massage, ultrasound, and functionally patterned strengthening exercises), we finally got around to a little walking. Oh, what a silent but elaborate tale walking tells.

Zoey had started using a cane over the past few weeks, so I really focused on her well foot and what she did with it. She claimed that she didn't walk like that normally and that the injury had altered her walk. I'm sure it had. Injuries do change the way you walk. But your Primary Movement Pattern still shines through, and hers projected a perfect picture of how her ankle problems all began.

Ankles are funny. They can bear weight in all sorts of contorted directions and handle odd exertions such as jumping and sliding into second base. They're a high-precision instrument designed with small but sturdy parts. When one of the parts gets blown out of alignment, however, others start to blow, too.

Little bones and ligaments and their intricate connections all depend on each other. And they can fool you. They can heal just enough to not hurt anymore, and they'll let you walk around without pain or a limp. But if you don't pursue a program of exercise and assiduous rehabilitation, your ankles can remain weak and become reinjured without much provocation.

Things get more critical if you have a predisposition to ankle vulnerability prior to any injuries. Both Zoey and her mom had amazingly long, skinny ankles. So because her mom had ankle problems, she thought she had a genetic ankle condition. But her ankle problem was not genetic.

Zoey had pronated feet, and that was what led to the majority of her problems. The similarities between Zoey's ankles and her mother's ankles were clearly evident, but it was a lack of strength that caused their ankle problems, not a structural defect. In fact, Zoey was very graceful, but she had a Primary Movement Pattern that included an outside heel strike, severe pronation, and foot turnout (plus, both feet crossed over her midline). She sat in her hips (which were also turned out), she held her chest high and breathed upward, her shoulder blades pulled back, and she held her head forward with her chin high, always appearing to look up a little.

Zoey was a take-charge person and very well-coordinated. She knew she needed to build ankle strength, and she took to her gait correction and exercise program like a duck to water. The hardest part was bringing her eyes, chin, and chest down. She wanted to "present" herself proudly to the world. Once she recognized that her new gait felt more comfortable, Zoey learned a new proud presentation.

We corrected her heel strike, and I had her do lots of Toes Feet/Feet Toes, along with Towel Scrunches and Alphabets. She loved doing Towel Scrunches at work (she was a set designer who worked as an artist all day—and yes, she worked barefoot sometimes). She said the Towel Scrunches were like worry beads. That exercise reminded her of a cat's kneading. She'd even pick up things off the floor with her feet, a great exercise to strengthen foot muscles. Zoey really dedicated herself to developing strong feet and ankles to prevent those irksome sprains. And she became equally committed to balancing the rest of her body.

Zoey did Semistraight Leg Raises, Standing Hamstrings, and Modified Mini-Squats to undo her hyperextended knees. She did Dial Outs, Hip Extensions, and Half-moons to give her hips strength and to reduce her tendency toward locking into external hip rotation (part of sitting in her hips). She stretched her piriformis and lower back muscles using the Supine Stretch Routine. She used the Table Exercise and the Double Knees to Toes for ab strengthening— with three pounds of weight on each ankle!

She did the Pec Stretch in a Doorjamb and both Scapular and Modified Push-ups to get her shoulders straight. She did Neck Flexors, Neck Extensions, and Side-Lying Neck Rotations to strengthen the muscles that kept her head back and her chin down. Watching her do the Slo-Mo Walking exercise was truly like seeing a Modigliani sculpture in motion.

Zoey defeated her ankle weakness. She also incorporated what she learned into her swimming to improve her strokes. She uses her abs much more, both in and out of the water. She has learned to stretch her pecs as she swims, she keeps her feet wider, and she kicks with her knees bent for more power. And her quads really get into the act as she holds her feet down as she kicks. She even holds her toes up as she gets out of the water.

Zoey's Personal Profile	Zoey's Gait Corrections	Her Exercises
inside heel strike, narrow base of support	center heel strike	Alphabet, Towel Scrunches, Toes Feet/ Feet Toes, Side-Lying Hip Circles
hyperextended knees	unlock knees	Semistraight Leg Raises, Standing Hamstrings, Modified Mini-Squats
sits in hips, weak abs and lower back	lift up and over	Dial Outs, Half-moons, Hip Extensions, Table Exercise, Double Knees to Toes, Slo-Mo Walking, Supine Stretch Routine
head and shoulders forward	pull head back, keep chin down	Pec Stretch in a Doorjamb, Scapular and Modified Push-ups, Neck Flexors, Neck Extensions, Side-Lying Neck Rotations

CONCLUSION

Walking is the most powerful creative tool that I know. It may be the most powerful spiritual practice known to man. Walking opens us up. Image by image, it feeds us so we can sustain our lives. In other words, we can walk our way out of a problem and into solution.

Julia Cameron, *The Vein of Gold*

The most powerful thing about this system is that it provides a process by which you can continue to unravel what isn't working and rebuild it with what does. It serves as a treatment for what's troubling you today, but that's just the beginning. You also have the means to eliminate future vulnerability to injury and pain, not to mention the perfect means to a healthy heart and lungs. You get to understand it. That's the real purpose of this book. It puts you in charge.

My learning curve is always changing. Sometimes I assimilate knowledge like a sponge, and at other times I wonder if I should be checked for Alzheimer's (actually, I call it Halfheimer's). I experience fluctuations in the way I pursue everything from spiritual development to sculpture. I've found that I'm at my best when I allow my inner rhythms to run their course. Forcing things has never worked for me. Recognizing this, I'm comfortable with experiencing magnificent spurts of growth right alongside the droughts. Both are equally instrumental to my productivity.

When you implement this system as a living process, you can sense how to pace yourself. Add a few corrections, let them sink in, strengthen up for them, and then rest. When it feels right, start again. Make it your choice. Yearning to experience a stronger body will fuel your progress naturally. You will not need discipline, only the desire to be physically in balance. If you learn to read your body and trust your instincts about it, that alone will make me feel that this book is a success.

It is my heartfelt prayer that each of you finds the way to wellness and an enjoyable walk.

APPENDIX A

GAIT CORRECTION AND EXERCISE FLOW CHART

Make a chart that outlines your first few weeks of gait corrections and exercises. List the first gait correction you've chosen to work on in one chart. On a separate chart, list the corresponding exercises you're going to do in support of that particular gait correction. You can use as many or as few corrections or exercises per week as you like (as was mentioned earlier, three corrections per week seems to be a good start). As you add more corrections and exercises to your program, the entire system (and the process of how you're getting there) will become more clear.

Study the sample charts below to give you an idea of how one person's program evolved. Notice that the gait corrections have corresponding exercises and vice versa. Sometimes an exercise will become too easy, in which case you may want to add repetitions or weight, or choose a more difficult exercise. Whichever way you upgrade, you'll still be working to reinforce a specific gait correction.

As you do the exercises, visualize how the strength or flexibility you're building contributes to that particular gait correction. Conversely, when you do the gait correction, recall how the exercise worked the muscles you need for that gait correction. This transposition process works both ways, between gait and exercise, exercise and gait, to help lock in the correction.

Remember, before you start your gait corrections, prepare by doing the following:

- Lift your body up and over, ribs down
- Unlock your knees
- Bring your weight to the front of your feet
- Bring your chest down and lower your chin
- Visualize widened steps and horizontal shoulder rotation
- Take a big sideways breath

Immediately following the two sample charts are two blank charts. Photocopy these charts, or create your own so you can make the chart bigger and easier to read.

Gait Correction Chart

Week 1	Week 2	Week 3	Week 4	Week 5	Week 6
Widen Step width 4.1	Pull heels out 1.2 Center heel Strikes 1.1	Lengthen Steps 4.3	Lengthen And Widen Steps 4.1 and 4.3	Long wide steps with heels out	Pull head up and back 8.0
Unlock Knees 3.1	Hold toes up longer 2.2	Point Knees outward 3.2 Leave heels down longer 1.3	Unlock Knees Headlight Knees down 3.1 and 3.2	Toes up longer Heels down longer	Lengthen Swing Phase
lift upper body, up and over 6.1	Breathe Sideways 6.2	Twist to face each Step 6.3	Move up & Over 6.1 Lengthen Swing Phase 4.4	Lift, twist and Breathe Sideways	Stay forward and Twist
	Use Your Arms 7.1	Move arms Straight through 7.3	Thumbs to front, Pinkies to rear 7.4	Use arms and Move them straight through	Thumbs to Front and Pinkies to rear

Exercise Chart

	Week 1	Week 2	Week 3	Week 4	Week 5	Week 6
	Side lying Straight leg raises (11)	Dial outs (9)	Hip Extensions (16)	Tray to Ceiling (16)	Modified Push ups (30)	Neck Extensions (34)
		Continue Semi-Straight leg raises (11)	Continue Dial outs (9)	Inner thighs (13)	opposite Arm & leg (18)	Neck Flexors (33)
	Semi-Straight leg raises (6)	Toes, feet Feet, toes (4)	Standing Sartorius (10)	Modified Mini-Squats (8)	Tip toes Walking (39)	Knee Extensions (5) THE Groucho MARX (38)
		Hip Flexors Sitting (17)	Calf Stretch (1)	Knee/Toe (12)	Heel walk (40)	
	Belly Press (21)	Belly Press with Sideways breath (37)	Oblique Crunches (27)	Standing Balance (20)	Cross Crawl (22)	Slo-Mo Walking (41)
		Alternating Knees (23)	Double Knees (24)	Table Ex. (25)	Standing balance	
		Cross Crawl (22)	Cross Crawl (22)	Back Shoulder Rolls (32)	Sitting LATS (29)	Back Shoulder Rolls (32)
I LIKE TO PUT MY STRETCHES HERE →	Press ups (8)	Supine Stretch routine (6)	Calf stretch (1) Hip Flexor Stretch (11)	Wall Stretch routine (5) Press ups (8)	Pec stretch in a Door Jam (3)	Supine Stretch routine (6) More Press ups (8)

Note: Be sure to correllate the exercises to the gait corrections. Use the exercise guidelines to determine numbers of repetitions and when enough is enough to go on. Beware of your goal for each exercise. Numbers refer to either Stretching/Strengthening exercises.

Gait Correction Chart

	Week 1	Week 2	Week 3	Week 4	Week 5	Week 6

Exercise Chart

Week 1	Week 2	Week 3	Week 4	Week 5	Week 6

APPENDIX B

BODY MOVEMENT AND MUSCLE ILLUSTRATIONS

Appendix B defines flexion versus extension, adduction versus abduction, and rotation. Muscle examples are provided, and often include several muscles that interact and contribute to a single movement (movements involve patterns of muscles that work in groups). A muscle chart follows (page 274) including a decoder table that identifies the function of each muscle.

FLEXION

Flexion is a movement that bends a body part, bringing an extremity closer into the body.

1. Neck flexion—brings chin to chest
   Muscle example—rectus capitis anterior, sternocleidomastoid
   Exercise example—Neck Flexors (when both muscles work together)
2. Elbow flexion—brings hand toward body (or toward shoulder or mouth)
   Muscle example—biceps
   Exercise example—Modified Push-ups (on the way down)
3. Knee flexion—brings foot toward bun
   Muscle example—hamstrings
   Exercise example—Standing Hamstrings, Modified Mini-Squats
4. Hip flexion—brings lower body toward upper body, or the reverse if feet are locked into place. (Note: Situps done with someone holding your feet use the hip flexors more than the abs.)

Muscle example—psoas

Exercise example—Hip Flexors

5. Shoulder flexion—brings arm over head

Muscle example—anterior deltoid

Exercise example—Cross Crawl

6. Trunk flexion—bends upper body toward your waist or vice versa

Muscle example—rectus abdominus

Exercise example—Low Ab Knee Switchers (also uses some hip flexors)

> For neck and trunk movement, flexion and extension are accomplished when the muscles on both sides of the spine work together. Rotation and lateral bends are accomplished by the same muscles, but acting only on one side, as directed by your brain.

EXTENSION

Extension is a movement that straightens and usually moves a body part away from the trunk.

1. Neck extension—pulls head up and back

Muscle example—splenius capitus

Exercise example—Neck Extensions

2. Elbow extension—straightens your arm

Muscle example—triceps

Exercise example—Modified Push-ups (on the way up)

3. Knee extension—straightens your legs

Muscle example—quadriceps

Exercise example—Semistraight Leg Raises, Knee Extensions

4. Hip extension—pulls your thigh or body back to a straight position from a bent one

Muscle example—gluteus maximus and minimus

Exercise example—Hip Extensions

5. Shoulder extension—another weird one; brings arm down from overhead or pulls arm straight back behind you

Muscle example—posterior deltoid

Exercise example—Cross Crawl

6. Trunk extension—pulls head back, curves body backward

Muscle example—erector spinae

Exercise example—Opposite Arm and Leg, Hands and Knees Balance

ADDUCTION

Ad in Latin means "toward." Adduction is the act of bringing body parts straight toward your center, or midline (the line that goes from your nose down through your navel to the floor between your feet).

1. Hip adduction—brings legs together

Muscle example—adductor magnus and longus

Exercise example—Inner Thighs

2. Shoulder adduction—brings arms down toward body

Muscle example—pec major and terres major

Exercise example—Modified Push-ups (while going up)

3. Neck and trunk do not adduct

4. Shoulder blade adduction—pulls blades in toward spine

Muscle example—rhomboids

Exercise example—Scapular Push-ups (while dropping down)

ABDUCTION

Ab means "away from" in Latin. Abduction is moving body parts away from your center.

1. Hip abduction—moves legs out or away from midline
   Muscle example—gluteus medius, tensor facia lata
   Exercise example—Side-Lying Straight Leg Raises and Hip Circles
2. Shoulder abduction—moves arms out from or away from your body
   Muscle example—middle deltoid
   Exercise example—not applicable to gait correction exercises, but
   the Standing Balance exercise uses the middle deltoid for holding
   the arms up and out, and Modified Push-ups use it for the lowering part of the exercise
3. Scapular or shoulder blade abduction—moves shoulder blades
   away from spine
   Muscle example—pec minor and serratus anterior
   Exercise example—Scapular Push-ups (the away part)

ROTATION

Rotation is a movement that turns or twists a body part.

1. Neck rotation—turns head to either side
   Muscle example—sternocleidomastoid, used on one side at a time
   Exercise example—Side-Lying Neck Rotations, Diagonal Neck
   Flexors
2. Trunk rotation—twists body to either side
   Muscle example—internal and external obliques
   Exercise example—Oblique Crunches
3. Scapular rotation—moves the shoulders
   Muscle example—*upward rotation*, upper trapezius and serratus
   anterior; *downward rotation*, pectoral minor, lower trapezius
   Exercise example—Scapular Push-ups

INTERNAL ROTATION

Internal rotation is a movement that brings an arm or leg in and around, toward the body.

1. Shoulder internal rotation—brings arm around and in toward the front and center
   Muscle example—anterior deltoid
   Exercise example—not applicable to gait correction exercises
2. Hip internal rotation—turns knee in
   Muscle example—gluteus medius and minimus
   Exercise example—Inner Half-moons

EXTERNAL ROTATION

External rotation is a movement that moves arm or leg out and around, away from body.

1. Shoulder external rotation—brings arm around and out toward the back
   Muscle example—posterior deltoid
   Exercise example—Modified Push-ups (the downward part)
2. Hip external rotation—brings leg around and out, away from the midline
   Muscle example—gluteus maximus, piriformis
   Exercise example—Knee/Toe, Outer Half-moons

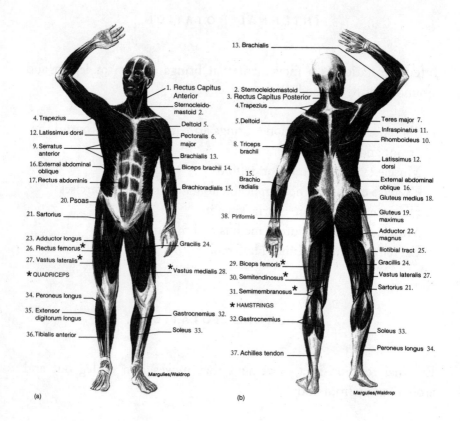

MUSCLE FUNCTIONS

1. Rectus capitus anterior—neck flexors
2. Sternocleidomastoid—neck rotators, flexors
3. Rectus capitus posterior—neck extensors
4. Trapezius—pulls head up and back, raises shoulders (a.k.a. "traps")
5. Deltoid—raises the arm away from the side (a.k.a. "delts")
   a. anterior—shoulder adduction and internal rotation
   b. middle—shoulder abduction
   c. posterior—abduction and external rotation

6. Pectoralis major—shoulder adduction (a.k.a. "pecs")
7. Teres major—shoulder external rotation
8. Triceps—shoulder and elbow extension
9. Serratus anterior—holds shoulder blades down
10. Rhomboids—pull shoulder blades toward spine (adducts)
11. Infraspinatus—shoulder external rotation
12. Latissimus dorsi—pulls shoulders down (a.k.a. "lats")
13. Brachialis—flexes elbow and brings hand inward
14. Biceps—flexes elbow and shoulder
15. Brachioradialis—flexes elbow with thumb up
16. External abdominal oblique—twists trunk
17. Rectus abdominus—bends body forward (trunk flexion; a.k.a. "abs")
18. Gluteus medius (a.k.a. "gluts")
    a. interior—twists leg inward
    b. hip abductor—moves leg straight out from midline
    c. exterior—twists leg outward
19. Gluteus maximus—hip extension and hip external rotation (a.k.a. "gluts")
20. Psoas—hip flexor (it's deep and barely visible on the illustration)
21. Sartorius—hip flexion and hip external rotation, knee flexion (a.k.a. "the Tailor Seat muscle")
22. Adductor magnus—hip adductor
23. Adductor longus—hip adductor
24. Gracilis—hip adductor
25. Iliotibial tract—flexes, abducts, and rotates thigh inward (a.k.a. "tensor fascia lata" or "TFL")
26. Rectus femoris—part of quadriceps, knee extensors
27. Vastus lateralis—part of quadriceps, knee extensors
28. Vastus medialis—part of quadriceps, knee extensors
29. Biceps femoris—part of hamstrings, knee flexors
30. Semitendinosis—part of hamstrings, knee flexors
31. Semimembranosis—part of hamstrings, knee flexors
32. Gastrocnemius—ankle extension, (a.k.a. gastroc plantar flexion with knee straight)

33. Soleus—ankle extension (plantar flexion with knee bent)
34. Peroneus longus—ankle eversion, pulls foot out
35. Extensor digitorum longus—toe extension, pulls toes up
36. Tibialis anterior—ankle flexor, ankle dorsiflexor (a.k.a. "anterior tib")
37. Achilles tendon—gastrocnemius and soleus join together to form the tendon that inserts into the heel bone (a.k.a. "gastroc tendon")
38. Piriformis—abduction and external rotation of hip

APPENDIX C

PAIN EVALUATION GUIDE

P ain, of course, is relative. People have different pain thresholds, so one would assign a 3 to a pain that another would assign a 5. You'll have to be the judge. Nonetheless, these guidelines and measuring tools can help you gain perspective as to whether outside help is advisable, and they give you a way to quantify your level of pain. Measuring pain is an important way to tell if your gait correction program is working. It also helps to indicate when you should worry about pain, or recognize it as a normal part of exertion.

There's an extremely tiny chance that a low level of pain indicates a problem that really requires further examination. But rather than become worried about minor pain, know that when a deeper problem exists, frequently there are additional symptoms other than pain.

To analyze your personal level of pain, you need to ask yourself these questions:

- How often does it come up? How intense is it, and does it vary in intensity depending on time intervals?

- What seems to bring on the pain? Does it seem to be getting worse or better?
- What do you find yourself doing to get rid of it, and does that always work?

Pain can be placed on a scale of 1 to 10:

1. A minor ache that is intermittent, perhaps more than a few times a week, but that does not stop you from doing anything. When you move certain ways, you notice it more, but it goes away as soon as you stop moving or sitting that way. You figure that if you ignore it, it will go away (often it does).

2. A deep ache that shows up more and more, but the pain doesn't stop you from normal activity. It shows up during certain movements, but over-the-counter pain relievers make it go away. You don't expect the pain to return because you have hours and even some days without it.

3. The same deep ache that comes and goes, but it's more consistent. Every day, for most of the day, the pain is there. You have reduced certain activities because of it. Pain relievers help, but you're still aware of the pain and you know that it needs attention.

4. The same deep ache lingers for part of the day but has flareups that are near impossible to ignore. During those times, it doesn't help to change positions, at least not right away, and rest slowly takes the pain away, with over-the-counter pain relief medicine. This level of pain may disturb your sleep if you roll into a certain position, but generally you sleep well.

5. Pain occurs several times throughout the day and can last for hours. On occasion it ruins your concentration and even your sleep. It's too deep for occasional pain relievers, so you take them all the time. The pain rarely goes away completely. It diminishes enough to allow you to manage your day, but it has a negative impact on your mood.

6. If you move gingerly, stay away from certain positions, and avoid certain activities, you're okay, although the pain is always there. You've graduated to stronger pain medication, and you still get shots of pain when you move the wrong way. You can work, but the drugs make you too fuzzy to drive. Your mood swings are palpable and you are tired from lack of sleep.

7. The pain exists all the time. You can barely function. The pain is too intense for drugs to help, and you can't concentrate on work. You manage to find some calm moments and can carry on a conversation even though you're distracted by the pain. Your sleep is a mess.

8. You're distracted by the pain all the time, and work is out of the question. You can manage at home, but even the pain medication sometimes doesn't help at all. You're tense and tired and having to work hard just to cope with the pain.

9. The pain is so severe that all you want to do is lie still and concentrate on breathing and resting so you don't tense up and magnify the pain. Some hours are worse than others.

10. There is no position and no relief no matter what you do.

If you have pain at level 1 or 2, you should monitor the pain and recognize that your body is trying to tell you something. Level 3 is your first big wake-up call. This level indicates that some form of action is definitely needed. Levels 4 and 5 are still manageable but require some objective analysis and care. Levels 6 and higher indicate that you should seek the help of a medical professional.

INDEX